D1063451

The Laying On of Hands

T. Ramsey Thorp, M.D.

For Eileen Murdoch

good luck

— T S Thorp

Hamilton Books
A member of
The Rowman & Littlefield Publishing Group
Lanham • Boulder • New York • Toronto • Oxford

Copyright © 2005 by
Hamilton Books
4501 Forbes Boulevard
Suite 200
Lanham, Maryland 20706
Hamilton Books Acquisitions Department (301) 459-3366

PO Box 317
Oxford
OX2 9RU, UK

All rights reserved
Printed in the United States of America
British Library Cataloging in Publication Information Available

Library of Congress Control Number: 2005929070
ISBN 0-7618-3249-1 (paperback : alk. ppr.)

∞™ The paper used in this publication meets the minimum
requirements of American National Standard for Information
Sciences—Permanence of Paper for Printed Library Materials,
ANSI Z39.48—1992

Contents

Contents

Acknowledgements

This work had been stimulated by years of doctoring, a legacy, my family, my peers and my patients. It is with deep gratitude that I wish to acknowledge them. Tilman Ramsey, M.D., my grandfather, practiced as a surgeon in Pineville, KY. While my contact with him was limited his greatest influence on me was through his daughter, my mother, Jane Ramsey Thorp. She had a keen intellect and was an energetic writer in her time. She was the Executive Director of the Northeast Mental Health Center in Philadelphia for a time. She was well aware of the difficulties in maintaining financial support of that center. My father, Francis Q. Thorp, M.D. was the principal influence in my direction as a doctor. He was cherished by us all and most certainly by his patients. His daily life was the beacon of my professional idealism. My wife Beth has been my continued support. She has been a motivator, a critic, an implementer. She helped me to focus and stay on target. It was her presence that really made this work possible.

LindaCarol Cherkin was my editor. She is no stranger to medical issues. She and I shared roots in northeast Philadelphia. While she was solid in her work as an editor I also felt that she believed in what I was trying to say. Her enthusiasm for the work was an affirmation for which I will always be grateful. I would also like to thank Lisa Kerber for her careful proof-reading.

I would like to thank those of my friends and peers who took the time to read the manuscript and give me constructive criticism and encouragement. David Mallery, my high school English teacher, was the first. It was really his first reading that gave me the sense to move on in the project. Jay Karfunkle, my neighbor and cohort in life, took pencil in hand and made me painfully aware of the need to find an editor. Henry Jordan, M.D. graduated with me from the University of Pennsylvania Medical School. His parents were classmates of my Dad's. We have been friends since 1958 and share many views concerning the evolution of our profession. John Kimberly, the Henry Bower Professor of Economics at The Wharton School at the University of Pennsylvania, has been involved in issues of health care policy and has indicated to me that this manuscript couldn't come at a better time.

My patients, so many of them, have encouraged this work, in particular N. Louis Shaten, Rev. William Guerin, and Rev. Paul Kennedy. It has been their compelling wish to have these views written. It has been a real joy for me to relate back to them, it has been done. I give my thanks to all of them.

Finally, the warmth of my family is a constant inspiration. To an individual they are the windows of my life. I am proud to mention that two of them have continued the legacy of love for medicine. Sons: Sheppard D. Thorp, V.M.D., Christopher R. Thorp, M.D., Benjamin S. Thorp, stepson Peter C. Paul, III; daughters-in-law: Kristen Wiley, Laura Cunningham, Maria Daniele; and grandchildren: Oscar, Mallory, Emma, Josephine and Cecily.

Individuals cited in this manuscript are all real; some have had their names changed to respect their privacy.

Relationship

"The patient-physician relationship is the heart of health care." Mike Magee, M.D. and Michael D'Antonio, The Best Medicine (New York: Spencer Books, 1999, 2003), 1.

I am writing this book to celebrate and savor the relationships that we have with one another. For a long period of time, I have been deeply concerned that we do not recognize that society is making it more and more difficult for us to establish connections with all those with whom we must relate—whether they are at home, school or business. And, perhaps this difficulty to connect has also developed internally within us.

As a physician, I am concerned that the once interactive doctor-patient relationship now has become so frail and almost non-existent. I do not believe that it is going to become any easier to nurture relationships given the direction our society is taking.

Therefore, the purpose of this book is to affirm the value of relationships; discuss their characteristics; how they are both established and threatened; and, finally, on what we need to focus to more fully realize our lives.

I grieve for the changes in these relationships, especially those that I have seen in the practice of medicine. My grandfather was a surgeon, my father a pediatrician. As a young man, I was exposed to the traditional doctor-patient relationship. While medical services to my father's patients were his first priority, the long hours my father spent

1

discussing the conditions of a patient with the family is still in my memory.

It was a "given" as to how much appreciation there was for the time and caring that was provided by the physician. Patients became better, not just because they received the correct care, but because they were being treated in a attentive, listening environment. There was something nurturing about it. The "Art of Medicine" is a well-known phrase and suggests some form of alchemy, beyond the technical, that is a necessary part of the medical armamentarium. During my early years in medicine, it was the mystery of the profession that attracted me to it.

Perhaps it is not "cool" in today's brisk, efficient society to foster the concept of caring. "Caring" can be viewed as soft and hazy in terms of our daily functioning. All of us prefer to believe that we are in control of ourselves. It is fascinating to listen to patients state their problems as if there should be simple solutions for perceived malfunctions. Common sense in many of these cases reveals areas of dysfunction in the day-to-day reality of their lives. Individuals being treated for high blood pressure often do not realize that, given the circumstance of their lives, increased blood pressure is a natural consequence of their environment and perhaps even from some of the choices they are making.

The human body is a remarkable barometer responding to the stimuli of its circumstances. For example, elevated blood pressure is often a signal of physiologic consequences to issues of stress, weight, and lack of exercise. One answer to hypertension might be medication. Another might be recognizing these issues in the larger context of a patient's life. Without acknowledging the underlying causes these individuals can be doomed to lives of chronic pharmaceutical management.

The "Art of Medicine" has to do with understanding the whole picture and not simply the numbers of the blood pressure reading. To achieve this end, there must be broad-based knowledge of the individual, the family and the environment. Given these parameters it is obvious that understanding the patient is critical. To this end, the relationship between the doctor and the patient is critical.

"Think about how much effort we put into finding just the right doctor and how much we value that connection when we make it. Then consider

how vital it is to have that relationship when a true crisis arises." Magee and D'Antonio, *Best Medicine,* 1.

"Behind closed doors, two individuals—one with a need and the willingness to trust, the other with knowledge and a willingness to respond —seek healing. They form a covenant of caring, a blend of science and humanity that is unique to the needs of one doctor and one patient at one time." Magee and D'Antonio, *Best Medicine,* 1.

Mrs. Lafferty

When asked, 'What is the essence of doctoring?' a soviet physician re-sponded, "Every time a doctor sees a patient, the patient should feel better as a result." Bernard Lown, *Lost Art of Healing* (New York: Zachary, Shuster, Harmsworth Agency, 1999), 88.

Mary Lafferty was in her eighties. Soft gray waves framed her pleasant full face. I had known Mrs. Lafferty and her husband for probably two decades. I had removed both of her cataracts and her husband's. Everything had gone well. Though her husband and been deceased for several years, Mrs. Lafferty was managing on her own. Her blue eyes had a twinkle to them and her smile was warm and welcoming. There was intelligence in her look, as well as a sense of nostalgia that was born from our shared experiences. Her last appointment was over a year ago and she had no new complaints to report.

Her first appointment had been in the seventies. Today she was a great grandmother, keeping up with her numerous children and grandchildren. She was taking good care of herself. Her weight was stable, she required some medication for blood pressure control and, while at times lonely, she was content with her life.

It had been a busy morning and I was about a half an hour behind. So, I apologized for keeping her waiting. Over the years my practice had become so busy that often it was difficult to stay on schedule. She graciously told me that she was fine, that she had reserved the morning for her eye exam and not to worry. First, I asked her if she had any

5

problems with reading or driving, questions to evaluate function. As far as she was concerned everything was normal. I asked her if she was able to maintain what she perceived as normal reading volume. This was fine. In my experience, even though patients are interested in their visual acuity, they are far more concerned about their level of function. One of the greatest challenges I have is assuring my patients of the functionality of reading. This involves not just the engagement of the eyes, but the intellectual process of reading. This also implied that factors leading to the success in reading were probably normal. The implication is that she has good general physical and psychological health. Admittedly, I am leading to my approach to my patient. I use this initial thought to suggest that I am not simply interested in the visual acuity, but of function. That is function of the eyes but also of the individual as a whole. I was fortunate with Mrs. Lafferty, as I knew her well and could bring her history to mind. By simply walking into the room, the first seconds with a patient are clues to so many things. A change in weight, slight pallor, strange body position, a mild tremor, even failure to make eye contact are all clues of issues that need to be addressed.

So far I had no sense of any significant issue or change. I asked if her eyes were comfortable, any dryness or itching? She gave a negative nod. Her refraction yielded no new information and her glasses were satisfactory. An evaluation with the slit lamp (a binocular microscope specifically designed for examination of the eyes) revealed well centered implants from her cataract surgery and normal intraocular pressure (a test for glaucoma). For examination of the retina, I used an eye drop to cause dilation of the pupils. After waiting for a few minutes, she returned for the last part of her exam.

The retina exam was performed and I found that her optic nerve and vessels looked fairly normal in both eyes. She did have a few small drusen in both maculas.

The macula is the most sensitive area of the retina. It is that part of the retina that gives us the ability to read; it is critical for all functions using central vision including driving, face recognition, and viewing television.

Unfortunately, sometimes within the macula, little yellow spots called drusen develop. Drusen may be small, discrete and flat. Sometimes they may be large, soft and poorly defined. In some cases there may be only a few; while in others there may be many. In many cases, vision may be unaffected by drusen and can even be stable for years. Multiple large drusen with soft margins have a poorer prognosis and can implicate the onset of loss of function.

Any change in the macula can be classified as maculopathy. This is a generic term and does not imply the most serious of all macular disease labeled macular degeneration. Macular degeneration is a term indicating a progression of disease leading to a loss of function described as "wet" (exudative) or "dry" (geographic atrophy).

In Mrs. Lafferty's case, she could be described as having maculopathy as indicated by the presence of drusen. She has been told of the changes in her retina. She has been told that the drusen that she has are of a more benign variety having a better prognosis. She does not have macular degeneration. Studies of small discrete drusen, such as hers, would suggest that she has a relatively low chance of developing macular degeneration. The risk of Mrs. Lafferty having her vision seriously affected is probably less than 10% throughout the rest of her life. This is important knowledge not only in how to support her in the care of her eyes, but also in the context of the strategies of her living situation.

The purpose of these observations is not to launch into a lecture about macular degeneration, but to discuss how Mrs. Lafferty's eye exam relates to her as a functioning human being. To be told by your physician that you are vulnerable to macular degeneration can be terribly destructive. Bernard Lown, M.D. in his excellent book "The Lost Art of Healing" discusses that words can maim. This is just such a case. There is an iatrogenic epidemic today relating to this disease entity.

Mrs. Lafferty is a comfortable, functioning woman in her mid-eighties. Life is good for her. What are my responsibilities to her as a doctor, scientist, healer? She can be told that she has macular drusen that could quite possibly develop into macular degeneration. As is typical in the community where I practice, many older individuals not only have heard of macular degeneration, but they also have acquaintances who are affected. They have a palpable fear of acquiring such a disease. It is also quite possible the small, flat drusen that she demonstrated may never cause a problem. The literature has reported that as few as ten percent of these lesions can lead to macular degeneration.

In my opinion, the purpose of my exam with a patient is to report the condition of her eyes and comment on any requirements either in the form of glasses, medication or surgery that might help maintain the health and function of her eyesight. I believe however, I have a further responsibility and that goes beyond the simple management of her eye condition. Patients want to be knowledgeable about their condition. They do not want to live in a state of physiologic doubt and fear. Finally, they do not want to lose control over their lives.

Dr. Edward Trudeau: "To cure sometimes, to relieve often, to comfort always." Lown, *Lost Art of Healing,* 319.

I want Mrs. Lafferty to be able to leave the office with a sense of comfort and understanding that her situation is not threatening and that it is being properly monitored and managed. I have real concern for patients who are abruptly told that they have macular degeneration and to return in six months for follow up. This is the kind of situation that needs to be reasonably discussed and put into context so that the patient has the tools to help adapt. Obviously, not all patients have the ability to absorb and process what may be discussed during an exam and a physician needs to be able to judge what is the appropriate approach to any given individual. We are not in the sole role of a diagnostician. Physicians should perceive their role as putting the patient in a position where healing is possible. How is this done?

Lewis Thomas: ". . . the capacity for affection, the essential element for healing." Lown, *Lost Art of Healing,"* 320.

In medical school we learn all the classic curricula. I have often enjoyed the statement, "In medical school I learned what was abnormal, it has taken me my lifetime to find out what was normal." How does one become a doctor? I remember passing my private pilot exam. After walking away from the plane my instructor said, "Well you passed the test; now go and learn how to fly." After graduating from medical school, now go and learn how to be a doctor.

". . . medical school . . . This is the beginning of a four-year intensive indoctrination aimed at instilling scientific competence, with little time

or effort being devoted to honing skills in interpersonal relations or in the cultivation of caring. The young physician is therefore neither interested nor trained in the art of listening." Lown, *The Lost Art of Healing,* 74.

In medical school there are no courses on intuition, trust, and communication. These characteristics would be considered a given? Medical school applicants are evaluated on more global issues with grades still being the great driver of acceptance. The purpose of this book is to talk about some of these innate qualities in rather specific terms. It is also a goal of this book to talk about barriers to healing in our current culture.

Pediatrician

My father was a pediatrician. He was a gentle man who loved people and people loved him. However, even more importantly, people trusted him.

During the Second World War, when few docs were around, he was the only doctor to take care of our busy neighborhood.

Since his office was located in the front of our house, I had the opportunity to watch him at work. Life in his office was very active. Today we would easily use the phrase 24/7 to describe his fulltime office hours which were often hectic. I don't believe there are many doctors today that can comprehend what it was like to practice medicine in those days.

Nothing was more important to my father than the welfare of his young patients. And, gaining their trust was paramount. Every decision he made in his practice was based on this principle. His belief was to maintain a strong bond with "his kids."

So, when "shots" were required, my father would miraculously disappear out of the examining room only to be replaced by the nurse who carried out the nasty deed.

He performed the exam in a small, simple, yet comfortable, room equipped with all the usual staples needed in a doctor's office. There were no dolls or stuffed animals. Back in those days, pediatric offices did not have much in the way of toys to increase the perception of child friendliness. It was up to my father to connect with his patients and make them feel comfortable.

As casual as it might have seemed to the untrained eye, even the exam was well-planned on his part. He would begin with the least offensive elements using the stethoscope to listen to the heart and lungs. He followed by palpating the abdomen; checking the neck and glands; taking the pulse and respiratory rate; all while studying the tone and color of the patient's skin.

After the gentlest aspect of the exam was completed, he hoped that some level of trust was achieved between the child and himself. Then, taking a delicate approach, he would look down the child's throat with a tongue blade and examine the ears with an otoscope.

During this entire time, he would be talking to the parent to try to pull out elements of the child's history that might be important. When all was completed, he would ask the family to bring the child to the front office where he would discuss the situation.

Dad's office was a special place. The first thing that you saw when you entered was his massive walnut desk. It was broad and covered with mail, patients' charts, a rack of pipes, family pictures and a tin of cherry tobacco. On the other side of the desk were two comfortable chairs for the family. As was his habit, Dad would meet with parents without the nurse present. This personal time could range from a few minutes to a more significant amount of time, depending on the needs of the family. Often he would light up his pipe and project the sense that there was nothing more important to him at the moment than his little patient and the concerns of the parents. It was during this meeting that the family would receive instructions and any necessary prescriptions. The constantly ringing phone in the background was handled by the nurse.

Dad started his career as a general family practitioner. Through the years he evolved, out of necessity and interest, into a pediatrician. Children and Dad were a perfect fit. In those days (1940's–1950's) he not only had a fulltime bustling practice, he delivered babies and also cared for the newborns in the hospital, as well. In addition, on Wednesday, Saturday and Sunday he made house calls.

Thus, I had little time to spend with my father. So, one of my tricks was to go on house calls with him. It gave us a chance to talk, but I can tell you I spent more hours in the car waiting and watching rain drops trickle on the windshield than in conversation.

His charges weren't high, in most cases less than 15 dollars paid in cash, check or barter. In 1958, at the peak of his earning power, my father made $30,000 which was a reasonable salary for the time. He sent my sister and me through private school, college, and, in my case, medical school.

In the later years of his career, he became keenly interested in exchange transfusions. This was an innovative treatment developed to be used on newborns with jaundice or those with blood incompatibilities with the mother. Dad enjoyed learning this new procedure, as he was challenged by the different form of mental activity required to do this quasi-surgical procedure. It was direct in its functionality; it had definable goals and measurable levels of accomplishment. And, for the first time in his long career he augmented his income by doing a procedure, thus increasing his ability to sense economic and personal freedom. He felt the rewards were measurable not just in terms of savings, but also in personal security. These thoughts he passed on to me as I entered medical school.

Medical School

Medical School was everything I expected. I had been prepped well.

Wearing the short white coat stiff with starch, we were filled with eager anticipation as we sat in musty lecture halls surrounded by portraits of former medical giants glowering down. The enthusiasm, the brotherhood, and the constant challenge of each new day filled all our lives.

The first two years of basic science kept us in the labs and offered us little in terms of patient exposure. The last two years were a deluge of clinical experience. During those years it was hard for any of us to believe that we would ever be able to complete any task satisfactorily, completely or comprehensively.

As third and fourth year medical students, we had to develop our own internal triage device to survive. It was important to develop a sense of priorities in managing the complex care of many individuals who were in the hospital at any one time. Unfortunately, I remember that one of our most outstanding and promising classmates was unable to complete his internship, because he never developed this indispensable skill.

I was part of the Vietnam generation and during my internship it was apparent that we would all be drafted. I learned that if I applied to the Navy's Flight Surgeon School, I would have some level of control over my life. I was accepted and sent to Pensacola, Florida and there I began a fascinating six-month tour with the Class of 104. We learned the physiology, psychology and practical matters relating to flight.

It was during this period and the two years assigned to the Carrier Air Group One that I had exposure to a wide range of clinical activities that allowed me to consider for my future the specialty of ophthalmology.

I leaned a great deal about myself during this period. The most important was that I truly enjoyed caring for people medically, psychologically, surgically, and even holistically. Thus, I knew I needed to find a specialty that would allow me to pursue all these interests.

Looking back, I know I made the right choice. Ophthalmology has given me all this. At the conclusion of my naval experience, I began my residency in ophthalmology. Once again, I experienced the same excitement I had when starting medical school. I was introduced to a new basic science, a new faculty, and a new brotherhood. After a six-month tour in the University of Pennsylvania Graduate School, the clinical program commenced. Three years later, I was prepared to open my office in the medical surgical practice of ophthalmology. It was July 1, 1970. This and the addition of another love, that of teaching, had come into my life. A requirement of my residency was to teach medical students. I took it on with a passion and this passion continues today. I consider teaching and sharing knowledge with such a gifted group of people who have dedicated their lives to medicine an enormous privilege.

Today's physicians might find my finances interesting. In 1970 when I started practicing, though my medical tuition was paid for, I was far from rich. My residency had compensated me to the point of $5,000 a year. My first office required a $30,000 bank loan. Malpractice insurance was nominal, a little less than a thousand dollars. My first secretary was a high school senior spending her summer months waiting to begin college. I remember in my first week of practice, I saw 20 patients . . . and most were family and friends.

A New Practice

In 1970 I found this new world of medicine exactly as I had hoped it would be. I was my own boss, with my own office and I looked forward to new challenges. I was married with three children under the age of six.

I had a very reasonable mortgage on our first home, and my chief financial concern was paying off my bank loan. I charged $20 for a complete eye examination and $400 for cataract surgery. Moonlighting became necessary to supplement the reality that my appointment schedule was not full. I scheduled four complete eye exams and two "briefs" each hour.

This is a striking comparison to today where our office charts number over fifty thousand patients. We have four ophthalmologists charging $125 for an eye examination and that $400 cataract surgery today costs $2000.

Even though today's waiting room is crowded and my schedule is booked three months in advance, I still feel good about the fact that I see the same number of patients each hour as I did when I first put out my shingle.

In 1970 when Medicare was five years old, other employee health-care programs had been in existence for some twenty years or more. Third-party pay was already a significant part of the medical environment. It was during this time, two changes occurred that were of significant importance to me and to my career.

First, I learned a new, rather aggressive ophthalmologist had opened his doors a few miles away and was charging twice as much as I was charging for an eye exam. It became apparent to me that the third-party would pay his fees. It was also apparent to me that there was no restriction from third-party payers to make up the difference. I realized I could then increase my charges with no financial pressure on the patient.

Secondly, I witnessed with admiration and awe, the building of a new, impressive eye institute. The hospital was the dream of one individual, his department, and the university. Within two years of its construction, a significant portion of the building became obsolete. This was mainly due to a technical advance in cataract surgery. The management of cataract patients was not required at the same level as it previously had been; therefore, 100 beds for post-surgical patients were no longer needed.

A few years later, this same sequence of events occurred at another famous eye institution. Thus, it became evident that healthcare delivery was changing so rapidly that strategic planning by both individuals and institutions required a new and innovative vision.

In 1970, when I started practicing, I made a decision that the critical features to my approach to patient examinations would be my priority and these identical features hold until today.

I had come from a very busy referral service where patients were cared for by technicians, assistant doctors and eventually by the chief of the department. I witnessed that these patients often seemed bewildered and cowered; some seemed angry by the lack of personal attention and concern. I knew then that this was not an outcome that I could tolerate. For this reason, I made the decision that I would only see my patients in a "one-on-one" setting. There would not be a host of other staff in the room. The initial part of the exam could be started by the technician, but the bulk of the exam would be completed by me and would be followed with time that I would spend with the patient discussing his or her case.

I believed that the examination room should be quiet and peaceful to encourage dialogue. I learned from one of my medical professors to try to discover something about my patient, beyond the simple scope of the medical encounter. His suggestion was to make a point of putting a note in the patient's record for "bonding" perhaps at a later visit.

Chapters of our Lives

Purpose: Writing the chapter titles of our autobiographies can help us appreciate the complexity and richness of our self-narratives. They can also help us to stand back and reflect from a distance and gain new perspectives.

Procedures: Take a few minutes to phrase or punctuate the flow of your life into discrete chapters or sections. Formulate a title for each, and write them on a sheet of paper, creating the *Table of Contents* for your life story.

Once written, reflect on the following questions that may interest you:

- How did you organize the flow of your self-narrative? (chronologically, event-based)
- How did you decide where to break the chapters? Did particular life events come into play here?
- When did you begin the story?
- When did you end the story?
- Does the change over time look more gradual or sudden?
- If the self-narrative were a novel, would it be a comedy, tragedy, history, mystery, adventure, or romance?
- What themes tie the chapters together? What conflicts are noted?
- Who is the primary author? Are there important co-authors that deserve credit (or blame!)?
- Who is the most relevant audience for this self-narrative? Who would enjoy it the way it is, and who would want to edit it?
- Are there any unwritten chapters? What has been left out? Who could validate it, and who could not?
- What would be a good title for your self-narrative? Is there some visual image or art that would capture the story better?

Losses often punctuate or organize life stories. When you story, it allows you to deconstruct, releasing y

Excerpted and modified from Neimeyer, R. (1998). *Lessons

on from boundaries... construct a

...g Loss: A guide to coping.

New York: McGraw Hill.

During this part of the exam, I believe it is essential for me to be seated. I can tell a great deal about my patients, their attitude, and, most importantly, their level of need. Obviously, there are cultural differences that must be addressed.

After taking a medical history and starting the eye examination, it is my custom to put drops in the eyes to measure for glaucoma. In doing so, I stand up and instill the drops while the patient reclines his or her head. After doing so, it has been my habit to gently pat the patient's shoulder to show a level of warmth and to acknowledge that I understand that no one likes anything put into the eyes.

"Lewis Thomas, in The Youngest Science, *comments wisely that touching is the oldest and most effective tool in doctoring. This statement rings true for me. I am persuaded that touching a patient provides advantages to the internist, as compared with the psychiatrist who sits removed and merely listens. Touching is a means for gaining significant insights. Frequently the conversation at a first interview is impersonal. The relationship with the patient often alters dramatically after the physical examination. The remoteness dissipates, supplanted by comfortable easy-flowing conversation. Material that was neither divulged nor suspected emerges without much probing. Questioning is no longer resented. A stranger a few minutes earlier opens up with intimacies usually earned only through long and trusting friendship."* Bernard Lown, *Lost Art of Healing* (New York: Zachary, Shuster, Harmsworth Agency, 1999), 23.

The basis for all these decisions is my belief in the importance of "one-on-one" and connecting mentally with the patient far beyond the scope of the eye exam itself. My sitting and establishing eye contact and even placing a hand on the shoulder, in my view, sets up an opportunity to deal with the patient, not simply as a health issue, but also as a human being.

Over 30 years later, I continue these basic principles in my practice. While they might appear relatively mechanical, I believe they provide an environment in which more subtle levels of communication can evolve.

"More than 90 percent of patients and doctors say their relationship is three things. It is compassion. It is understanding, based on active

patient education. And it is partnership with shared decision-making."
Mike Magee, M.D. and Michael D'Antonio, *The Best Medicine* (New
York: Spencer Books, 1999, 2003), 3

   *Dr. Jing-Bao Nie, "Science treats all human beings alike, ignoring
dissimilarities to find common features. Medicine must follow science,
of course, but it also follows humanities, since a humanistic approach
treats every individual as a unique person. This relationship appears totally secular, but there is sacredness in it."* Mike Magee and D'Antonio,
The Best Medicine, 6.

   *"Just as patients are not interchangeable, neither are physicians.
Aside from their differing cultures, personalities, and life experiences,
they differ in skills and in their willingness to consummate relationships
and balance technological and human concerns. All of which is to say
that matching a patient to a physician is a highly individualistic and extraordinarily important concern." Mike* Magee and D'Antonio, *The Best
Medicine,* 6.

While certain elements of the practice of medicine were meant to be
a stable part of the "product," innumerable changes did occur. We became busy and thus space requirements developed. Staff needed to
be expanded. Overhead increased with all its attended consequences.
The technology of medicine progressed exponentially. The requirements of healthcare payers became more invasive. Bureaucracies
evolved establishing many laws delineating expectations.

   More serious, but perhaps more subtle, were the cultural changes in
the manner of trust, accountability and professionalism. During the
halcyon days of my father and grandfather, the physician was considered, perhaps euphemistically, beyond reproach. Not so today. The
medical environment has become progressively toxic to the point that
in Pennsylvania this year (2004) we have had some 5 percent of our
physician community quit, retire or move out-of-state.

   In fact, many physicians do not encourage their children to follow in
their footsteps and choose medicine as a career. Remembering back to
my own childhood, being a physician was the only occupation that I
conceived that I wanted to do. Medicine, like some other professions,
invites an individual to enter into a constructive relationship with another human being in which the outcome benefits both participants.
This is done in such a way that the recipient's expectations are met not

only by the talents of the deliverer, but to some extent through his or her altruism.

The true professional puts the interests of the client above the personal interest of himself. Altruism never occurs in a vacuum. I am talking about a relative level. It has been said, "If there is no margin there is no mission." This certainly applies here.

"The AMA states that 'medicine is a special kind of human activity— one that cannot be pursued effectively without the traits of humility, honesty, intellectual integrity, compassion, and effacement of excessive self-interest.'" Mike Magee and D'Antonio, The Best Medicine,4.

In my experience, physicians benefit in more ways than simply making money.

Many retiring doctors have said that they missed going to work as they had no idea how much their practices had meant to them. They felt in some sense their own need to be involved in this unique doctor-patient relationship.

The following is a series of doctors' comments about their practices and patient relationships. They are from Dr. Mike Magee and Michael D'Antonio's book *The Best Medicine.* They are truly insightful.

"As a whole, my patients have taught me that I must be a human being first, and then a doctor." 23.

"I focus pretty intently on taking both a social history and medical history. I take my time and listen, because in that information are some important clues to what a patient is feeling. Few patients are going to put everything out there for you. You have to intuit some things, and use your experience to ask the right questions." 37.

"It's much easier to deal with things if you let yourself feel what is going on. You also get much more information from your patients if you reveal yourself as a person." 45.

"It wasn't the surgical success that was the most important thing. It was that we helped that young man stay whole as person with a future." 61.

"You figure out how to approach families based on the context of their lives. I'm not talking about their medical history. It's how they live. I used to be much tougher about things, before I understood what the context meant." 123.

"I think the advice I would give other doctors who want to have a good relationship with their patients is that they let themselves enjoy the time they spend with people." 166.

"How do I work on the relationship? By being myself and not running away from the emotions in the situation." 171.

"The credibility comes from the quality of care we provide the community." 172.

"That's what you get out of investing in your relationship with families. They let you into their lives, and you learn a lot about how to live your own. It's something that benefits me more than anyone. It keeps me from burning out. It keeps me from getting out of balance with my own life and my own problems. It is why I am in medicine in the first place and the key is not to forget it." 173.

"In this situation I try to build on three qualities: trust, respect, and 100 percent honesty. I don't have to write very detailed notes about what I did or didn't tell a patient because I know that I always tell everything I can as soon as I know it." 192.

"At the time I had been talking a lot about the fact that the human side of medicine, the emphasis on patients and doctors relating compassionately was dying. We were making great technological advances: new medicine, new machines, new procedures. But we were losing touch with how to ease suffering, how to connect." 195.

"One of my messages is that in these relationships with patients we get all of the unexpected, exciting things that make life enjoyable. Every interaction we have with a patient or family is an opportunity for an adventure. So many things happen because we open ourselves up to others." 195.

"The first thing I do to try to make the relationship real is teach them to complain. I tell them that I don't know what it's like to be the patient, to have cancer. It's a matter of control. Patients often feel like they have lost control of everything. I try to give it back." 202.

Dialogue

Dialogue between the patient and the physician should be a given. There should be a connection between the physician and the patient that is always open, honest and comfortable. In most situations, involving the patient's personal history and medical care, this connection does occur. With regard to fees or payment for services, doctors have not been forthcoming. It has been my experience, that this has been a "zone of no communication". I can understand the reticence, but it mystifies me why either participant seems unwilling to open the conversation.

Prior to third-party payers it was the responsibility of the doctor to indicate the cost of the services to the patient. The doctor could do this directly or through one of his/her staff. Depending on the patient's ability, fees were adjusted and courtesy was applied as cases warranted. If a patient was not able to pay, the doctor was immediately aware of the situation and thus he or she was able to make a modification.

Professional courtesy was always "understood," and considered to be a part of the culture. Individual physicians might vary to whom they would offer courtesy. Typically professional courtesy would be given to family, close friends, perhaps neighbors, clergy, and other doctors and their immediate families.

In the late forties, with the advent of third-party pay, the economic conversation between physician and patient became more complicated. This was further compounded by the launch of Medicare in 1965.

Medical students are not prepared for the economic realities of running a practice. In 1970, I set my fees by what was commonly charged in the community. As I have said, I learned one of my earliest lessons when my new competition in the area charged twice as much as I charged and received greater return without question, from the third-party payer. After giving it consideration, I saw no reason why I couldn't do the same. When I did raise my rates, to my surprise, there was no objection from either my patients or third-party payers. From that time on until present, I have made a point of addressing my fee schedule. It seemed to be the appropriate thing to do. There was no opposition from the payers. I continued my practice of courtesy discounts as an integral part of the professional culture in which I was raised. I believed this consideration a quality of my profession which was sacred and of which I was quite proud.

Most physicians in my generation wanted to be their own boss. There is a desire to have a sense of control over day-to-day activities. The doctors' decisions could be influenced by the patient, to some extent, and by the staff and perhaps by peers. However, it was the physician who was in control of his or her own economics with no bureaucratic regulation. Thus, if a physician was irresponsible, he or she generally wouldn't be as busy, necessitating him to change his or her behavior. As third-party payers evolved, controlling physician clinical and economic behavior became a prime objective.

In the mid-seventies, I became aware of a "physician profile" which was compiled by the payers as a result of a physician's billing activities. It became apparent that I had to address this "profile" annually in order to maintain my anticipated level of revenue. This was a conversation I had with the payer and never with the patient. In the early years it also became apparent that revenues coming from the new "profile" charges did not meet my expected levels. Charges and revenues were two different items altogether. This pattern evolved at the institutional level and exists to this day. Patients often relate stories about their outrageous hospital bill, and are surprised to learn that the hospital actually only receives a portion of those charges. In a sense two different accounting books are being maintained, one for charges and the other for revenues.

All these financial arrangements are handled without the patient being involved. In the grand schemes of strategic planning and basic budgetary mechanics it is highly complicated if not impossible. Note again that there is no patient input into this dialogue. It almost seems humorous at this point to wonder if there are any considerations of professional courtesy in this architecture.

> *"To navigate successfully around the shoals of the healthcare system demands extraordinary insight, skill, patience, and forbearance. In the present environment of managed care, even these admirable qualities may not prove sufficient."* Bernard Lown, *Lost Art of Healing* (New York: Zachary, Shuster, Harmsworth Agency, 1999), 320.

The patient is sometimes brought back into the loop when the insurer must raise premiums to cover increased costs. Unfortunately, often the patient is still masked from the situation, as generally the insurer is not paid by the patient, but by the employer. Thanks to labor movement in the forties, healthcare benefits were seen as an alternative to increasing wages and since that time employers are one of the first groups to feel the added pressure of rising healthcare costs.

For several reasons, patients were eventually involved with their co-pay arrangements. It was felt that this would give them some sense of accountability in the use of services and, more importantly, it would reduce the costs to the employers. It was readily apparent that patients did not like co-pay arrangements and found that secondary insurance was necessary. Much to their distress, particularly for Medicare patients, co-pay policies have become almost prohibitively expensive.

Since the forties, healthcare has progressed from a patient's privilege to his or her right. This cultural fact influences the office environment and alters the professional tone. It is an unintentional consequence of the destructive nature of a complex economic environment. If the two key players involved, the physician and patient, do not have a direct economic interface, they will lose control over their relationship.

Hence, my reasons for discussing this subject at this juncture. My ability to relate to my patient is dependent on our having a rational understanding of the economic consequences of our needs for one another. It would appear that both the patient and I have suffered attenuation so severe that there is little attention given to either the specifics of the charge or the manner in which it is paid.

At this stage in my practice in most cases I am only allowed to see a patient if they are referred to me by their primary doctor.

Now, here is the logic of the HMOs. After having been in practice for over three decades, I find it somewhat bewildering that my HMO patients are required to have a referral slip from their primary doctor to see me, a physician whom they have known for many years. I have had situations in which the primary doctor is unknown to the patient and yet I have known this patient and family for three generations. Still, according to HMO regulations, the patient cannot be seen by me without that all-important referral.

Without this referral, I will not be paid by the HMO. The HMO has also said that in some instances I cannot (categorically) see the patient.

Again, what is the patient's participation in this situation? And, as a professional, what can I do to facilitate what sometimes is a frustrating situation for both patient and physician? How can I act as the professional that I have been trained to be and know I am?

Continuity of care is also at risk in this scenario. Traditionally, continuity has been a mainstay in the practice of medicine.

"Contrary to common belief, patient-physician relationships in America were surprisingly long-term. About 80 percent of patients had relationships with their doctors for an average of seven years. And nearly 30 percent had been with the same doctor for more than ten years. The patient-physician relationship is the heart of health care." Mike Magee, M.D. and Michael D'Antonio, *The Best Medicine* (New York: Spencer Books, 1999, 2003), 2.

Only time will tell if this will continue in our current medical climate.

Practical Lessons

I learned one of my most valuable lessons when I served with the United States Navy's Carrier Air Wing One. I spent almost two years as a flight surgeon on the Carrier Franklin D. Roosevelt (CVA-42) along with 40 other corpsmen.

Our admin was a remarkable officer who was prime for the job. His name was Lt. James Dewhirst. "Dewey" was an outstanding role model who had worked his way up through the ranks. One of the most significant lessons I learned from working under him was to be responsive to principles of service. Medical training really never engages in this specific doctrine. In the day-to-day practice, however, it became an obvious priority.

Ever since being introduced to the principles of service from Lt. Dewhirst, these concepts have been important to me. Service should be the most essential objective for any industry, including medicine. Thus, I have always believed that the patients desire, deserve, and should receive good service. The ability to build a medical practice is directly related to the quality of service that has been provided.

In my office, I have identified specific priorities that include: being on time, being accessible, providing top quality medical services and doing so with reasonable fees. These continue to be what I believe are the fundamental concepts to providing good service to my patients. In 1970, when I started my medical practice, I was able to fulfill these goals. In today's medical culture, I find there are challenges to complete these expectations.

One problem is that a doctor's productivity is limited by the amount of available time he has to see his patients. There are only so many hours in the day to work. Many doctors utilize Physician Assistants within their practices thus allowing more patients to be seen per unit of time. Physician Assistants are giving doctors more time by taking medical histories and performing some physical examinations. Competent work can be done within such a system and may even lead to greater efficiency and productivity; however, if the doctor-patient relationship is supposed to be to be a necessary part of total service received then that aspect of care most certainly will suffer.

With increased attention given to third-party payers, most office staff is preoccupied with administrative details. Often a patient is perfunctorily greeted by the fleeting glance of the receptionist who then instantly returns her eyes to a computer terminal. Patients walk through the door expecting to find solutions to their problems. The first question they are asked has nothing to do with their health, but about their insurance. Even though this attitude may be more accepted by patients as a requirement to running an efficient office, it is off-putting and there is no doubt that the doctor-patient relationship suffers.

Today, the patient, the doctor, and even medical services are considered commodities. With recent federal regulations this process will continue to evolve. These changes will continue to force the evolution of care. Healing is not even identified as a recognizable product. Professionalism is an anachronism. As the physician is regarded less by patients as a central part of the healing process, these patients will feel anxious about the level of service that is available to them. Whereas in the past the physician had been a listener, diagnostician, therapist and healer; now in this new roll he or she has been relegated to simply that of a mechanic. A diagnosis can be determined and appropriate solutions prescribed, end of story.

> *"Treating differs from healing. The former deals with a malfunctioning organ system, the latter with a distressed human being."* Bernard Lown, *Lost Art of Healing* (New York: Zachary, Shuster, Harmsworth Agency, 1999), 99.

It is important to distinguish between disease and illness. A good metaphor is that posed by Bill Moyer:

You're driving the car and you see flashing lights in your rear view mirror. There is a police car behind you. You wonder if they are trying to pull you over for some infraction. You begin to worry, you perhaps sweat a bit, the heart rate changes, you become anxious. Slowly the police car advances and then passes you moving on forward and proceeding after someone in front of you. You suddenly feel a warm rush of relief.

Disease defines the condition. Illness is how you feel about the disease. In the metaphor there was an illness without disease.

As doctors we are responsible to deal with disease and illness. Healing cannot occur without addressing both. Doctors can, if not attentive, aggravate both. If we do not attend to illness the disease can be accelerated.[1]

The physician has handed over his roll as a healer. There isn't enough time for him/her to provide such service and frankly the insurers don't care.

There is already evidence that the patient has recognized the problem and is developing alternative healthcare modalities. Patients are very sophisticated and are researching lifestyle issues, exercise opportunities, and better nutrition to achieve immediate remedies to many of their health problems. Alternative therapies such as yoga, acupuncture, massage are pursuits that are common for today's patients. And, let's not forget the internet. The savvy patient can "surf the net" and visit the myriad medical sites and even "google" specific medical subjects.

"People everywhere are starved for meaning, purpose, and spiritual fulfillment in their lives. To lead healthy, full lives, we require a positive sense of meaning, just as we need food and water, for without meaning life withers." Larry Dossey, M.D., *Reinventing Medicine (San Francisco:* Harper Collins, 1999), 11.

Many patients are assuming responsibility for their own well-being. This is both reasonable and satisfactory until there is a threat to their health. At this point, there is a need for medical intervention and the full elements of service will apply at this critical juncture. This is where a physician, with whom you have developed history, can successfully intervene. And as the patient, you will want that physician to know you and to know all about you. You will want him or her to care for you and to guarantee that the appropriate functions that you require will be completed. And, finally you will want to feel that you are being cared for in the correct manner and that you are not subject to inexorable financial risks.

Ultimately we are all going to need to see a doctor. My prayer for all of us is that the physician who is waiting to treat us will have those qualities I have described.

Along with service, continuity is also one of the most critical components of successful healthcare. Unfortunately, like service, continuity is an issue not approached in medical school. After three decades of practicing medicine, I see the extraordinary value of continuity. Continuity is not a question of simple loyalty. It is an issue of profound significance in understanding how patients function. Blood pressure can vary day-to-day and in different levels of stress. After knowing someone for ten years, a physician is in a much better position to know how to handle the situation. In an ironic battle with the HMOs and the patient's desire for choice, there has been an argument brought forward on continuity of care.

Mrs. Lafferty has macular drusen and has a potential risk for macular degeneration. She is otherwise in good health, lives alone and is happy with her life. If I send her to a retinal specialist for further evaluation what will become of her? Most probably, she will be told that she has the earliest evidence of macular degeneration, and since her eyesight is at risk, she should be followed closely. She will be given a piece of graph paper to use as a check for any deviation of central vision in the hope that they might stabilize the process. And, finally, she will be advised to return in six months.

If she is troubled with this diagnosis, she will seek a second opinion. And, most likely, a second opinion will give her the identical diagnosis. Mrs. Lafferty is now faced with the fear that, as an 83-year-old living alone, she may have to seriously consider altering a lifestyle to which she was accustomed or in which she was comfortable. For example, she may not be able to drive, if there is a possibility that she may lose her central vision. She may have to sell her home and consider moving into a retirement community. If her ability to read is taken away, what will Mrs. Lafferty do to sustain herself? Many thoughts are swirling or spinning in her head. She remembers friends who became severely depressed when they lost their vision. In fact, she isn't sure if macular degeneration would mean that she is going blind.

How has Mrs. Lafferty been served? How has she been healed? Where is the continuity in her treatment? This is a wonderful happy woman in what should be a potentially marvelous period of her life.

The challenge that the physician should welcome is the opportunity to manage Mrs. Lafferty's condition by giving her every opportunity to live out her days happy and complete. Isn't this why we chose medicine?

"Effective patient management requires appreciation of the art of healing, in which one is guided by experience, by the recall of a similar case, and by the exercise of common sense. A sense of humility, too, is an asset, for any prescription or advice has a substantial measure of conjecture. Much medical data is increasing based on epidemiological studies of large populations. A doctor, however, confronts a single, singular individual. There is never any certainty as to where the individual fits on the normal statistical distribution curve. Statistics may present probabilistic truth, but they shroud souls and obscure individuality. When confronting uncertainty, the physician has to be an ombudsman for the patient. But advocacy requires caring. Only then can the physician somehow surmount the agony and absurdity of human decision." Bernard Lown, *The Lost Art of Healing,* 119–120.

Macular Degeneration

Macular degeneration, the leading cause of irreversible loss of a patient's central vision, continues to be a huge public health issue, especially for the elderly population. It is predicted that the United States population over 65 will increase 63%, from 16.6 million in 2000 to 27 million in 2005. And, some five percent will develop macular degeneration, presenting an enormous challenge for our society.

The research in treating macular disease is prolific. Prevention has been one avenue of approach. Risk factors can be modified by a healthy diet with relatively high doses of vitamins C and E, zinc and beta carotene. Low fat intake may be helpful. Recent reports suggest lower risk with high intake of fish and nuts[2]. Smoking is a risk factor. Therapy for macular disease has included laser treatment to the retina, enhanced laser with photo dynamic chemical called Verteporfin, radiation, transpupillary thermotherapy, surgical translocation of the macula and newer medications aimed at abnormal vascular proliferation in the macula. It is not the purpose of this discussion to go into any of the details of the research process. It is important to acknowledge the healthy pursuit of a dependable course of management for macular degeneration.

With all the attention given to macular disease, doctors have not discovered the "silver bullet." Macular degeneration is irreversible and incurable. Patients diagnosed with the disease are told that their vision will slowly decrease. At best therapy is palliative. The attempt is to maintain the size of their central blind zone so that it does not expand. Diagnosed patients are often frail and have difficulty making decisions. They are frightened, feel disempowered and are frequently depressed and it is a challenge to advise and comfort them. When their vision does not improve, most patients are disappointed. Their only solace is that their sight may stabilize and they may enjoy some sense of better peripheral vision and better contrast.

Research must use clinical trials to validate the effectiveness of these treatment modalities. These are the necessary tools for advancing our knowledge. Studies have been very beneficial in evaluating both the advantages and disadvantages of specific treatments. There is exceptional investment involved as the potential market for satisfactory remedies is significant. Clinical trials must be established to assure that there is not a conflict of interest between researchers and pharmaceutical providers. The FDA must bear the responsibility for the means in which these products are brought to market. This has been fraught with difficulty. Recent discussions have focused on the desire to "speed" new drugs to market. The FDA has been unable to fund the researchers needed to keep up with the demand for assessing new drugs, as well as evaluating medications already on the market.

A recent debacle concerning the CMS (Center for Medical Service) and the FDA evolved out of clinical trials for photodynamic therapy (PDT), a treatment for macular degeneration. It is an interesting case, as it shows the complicated nature of how bureaucracies perform. PDT had been used with some success for exudative lesions of the macula. Clinical trials of occult lesions had not been convincing. Anxious doctors and fearful patients had put a lot of pressure on CMS to approve the treatment. CMS eventually acquiesced without FDA approval. Photodynamic regimen was then applied throughout the United States. PDT is expensive and may require several treatments. The elderly were unable to support such expensive care and were grateful for CMS support, as were the doctors. CMS reversed its position six months after it had approved the treatment. The reasons given were the failure of a one-year clinical trial and the position of the FDA. It was back to square one both for the researchers and the anxious and confused patients. The dialogue among the CMS, FDA, researchers, and pharmaceutical companies is an interesting piece of theater. I think this shows some of the vulnerability of complex governmental organizations. Accountability becomes vague and errors can occur.[3]

One of my concerns in the treatment of macular degeneration is the result in the management of the disease. Sadly, to date, there is no cure, only palliation which is difficult to measure objectively. Many patients are often not able to perceive a difference. Of major long-term concern, will be the costs of such therapy. In a healthcare industry with progressively constrained resources, can we envision the treatment of such a disease with laser applications every three months at a cost of several thousand dollars, especially given the uncertain outcomes? If there is no "silver bullet," how do we decide on the best management, in the caring of such a difficult issue?

A recent article by Paul Sternberg, M.D. in the American Journal of Ophthalmology gives interesting insight into the problem:

> "*From our perspective, photodynamic therapy remains the best currently available, approved treatment of neovascular age-related macular degeneration. Unfortunately, it only benefits a modest subgroup of patients with overall disappointing results. There is rare improvement in vision, many patients describe a steady decline in vision, and there is often some degree of patient disappointment and dissatisfaction.*" Paul Sternberg and Hilel Lewis, "*Photodynamic Therapy for age related macular degeneration: a candid appraisal,*" American Journal of Ophthalmology, volume 137, issue 3 (March 2004): 483–485.

As a further concern, Dr. Sternberg warns of conflicts of interest:

> "*As new therapies for [age-related macular degeneration] AMD and choroidal neovascularization enter the market, it is essential that we maintain professional and scientific integrity in the conduct of clinical trials and impartiality in the reporting and interpretation of their results. Stricter guidelines regarding the roles of physicians, pharmaceutical companies, and other parties with significant interest in clinical trials may help to optimize patient benefit, minimize waste of healthcare resources, and preserve the integrity of our profession.*" Sternberg and Lewis, "*Photodynamic Therapy,*" 483–485.

A lead editorial in the New York Times reinforced this concern. The FDA has an obligation to clear conflicts of interests when judging the merits of a drug. "The deeper problem is that links between drug companies and medical researchers are pervasive. Unless the FDA makes a more aggressive effort to find unbiased experts or medical researchers start severing their ties with industry, a whiff of bias may tint the verdicts of many advisory panels."[4]

We are dealing with a frightened population with devastating changes in their lives with treatment programs that are expensive and offer only palliation. There is an enormous need for professional and human oversight.

Trust

"To heal requires a relationship marked by equality—a key element in a sound doctor-patient relationship—and reciprocal respect. This is not automatically granted by either; it needs to be earned. Without respect, a doctor cannot gain a patient's trust. Respect is not the mush of language. As the essayist Anatole Broyard, dying of cancer, commented about his doctor, 'I don't trust anyone who tells me that he loves me when he doesn't even know me.' The patient desires to be known as a human being, not merely to be recognized as the outer wrappings for a disease. Only the patient is capable of widening the doctor's focus to encompass the larger domain of the person who is ailing. Therein resides the art." Bernard Lown, *Lost Art of Healing* (New York: Zachary, Shuster, Harmsworth Agency, 1999), 313.

In the spring, as medical school students our thoughts turn to commencement and to the beginning of a new era. It is the time of personal accomplishment and the satisfaction of a job well done. No matter how many commencements or graduations I attend through the years I always have a sense of reverence for tradition, for commitments made and for expectations that have been met. On graduation day, these three principles are gloriously clothed in cloak, gown, with special hoods indicating the degree earned.

Elgar's Pomp and Circumstance resonates as the notables ceremoniously process. A sense of awe and unquestioned respect fills the air. During commencement we recited the Hippocratic Oath: Primum Non

Nocere, *first do no harm.* There was a sense of the sacred commitment
of the doctor for the well being of the patient. This was couched in
the quiet sanctity of graduation from medical school. Surrounded by
respected faculty, friends and family, the new doctor assumes an extraordinary sense of responsibility.

There is no course on trust in medical school; no examination or final grade, yet it is one of the most important components of becoming
a physician. Trust can be earned and can foster relationships. Trust
doesn't come with a label, but can be sensed. In high school I worked
on a farm for several summers. As a city boy this was a wonderful opportunity for me to experience a different culture and to enjoy a new
way of life. One of the earliest experiences I had was working with
the animals. I quickly learned that I was more comfortable handling
horses, for example, than geese. I witnessed that the farmer had an exceptional level of comfort and ease with the various animals. There
was respect, caring and communication. "Horse Whisperer" is a good
example of the level of connection that might occur in the best of
circumstances. While this comparison may seem a bit far-fetched, it
applies, as well, to medicine and to the level of trust that must exist
between the patient and the doctor for the relationship to be successful
or thrive.

Trust must be earned. It also must be cultivated. When the bond of
trust is broken it becomes very difficult to rebuild. Trust can be recon-
structed, but it may take time and the process of repairing that bond can
be quite sensitive.

Trust is an unspoken agreement of permission between two persons
or among people. It is the opening of vulnerability. It assumes that one
individual is comfortable to the extent of vulnerability. He or she
agrees to "partner" in a decision or act. There is a synergy of will.
There is a permission to work together. With this, the relationship can
build on a new level of collaboration. It is hard to define; however,
there are characteristics that allow an individual to sense that he or she
is in a trusting relationship. There may be the satisfaction in the real-
ization of a successful outcome.

There should be a sense that we are invited into this partnership.
Sudden changes in behavior do not favor the evolution of trust. Surprise is not an inducement for trust. In fact, surprise is a risk factor to

any trusting relationship and might mean that a basic mutual understanding was never in place.

Continuity is an aspect of trust, as evidenced by a positive relationship that has extended over a long period of time. Trust is much more difficult if not impossible given a short term of exposure. A trusting feeling can be evident immediately, but it takes time to prove itself.

Cultural and ethnic differences and language barriers can obviously complicate the picture. That brings me back to the farmer. I find it fascinating to recall his ability to manage a wide variety of animals and their needs. My son, a veterinarian, also has to deal with various sets of needs as did my father, the pediatrician. Both had to develop trust with their patients, be they helpless animals or children. Their approaches were the same—no surprises, patience and a sense of partnering.

Launching a medical practice, after being nurtured in the medical school environment, requires cautious introspection. Our current culture is not a trusting one. In my naiveté I assumed that I would have been able to establish the doctor-patient relationship without much difficulty.

I watched my father enjoy a very satisfactory reputation based on the continuity of long and trusting relationships with his patients. So, during my first months in practice I was fortunate to have as patients, individuals with whom I had some previous connection. My first patients included my family and friends; neighbors; classmates and ultimately referrals. Referrals were, and still are, a wonderful help in expanding my practice, as these new patients were recommended to me by someone who also had trust in me. There was the assumption through these patient-doctor relationships that I was trustworthy. "Word of mouth" was the typical manner in which practices grew. One satisfied patient led to another. In the first year, I had accumulated one thousand new patients. The practice continues to grow at about that rate every year.

Trust between my patients and myself was always an objective. I have worked hard to be able to say that it has never appeared to be a problem. The way of life around us, however, continues to change. It is those vital elements of trust that I believe are being undermined. The societal assumption today is that we are not trustworthy and, therefore, instruments must be provided to assure trust.

Let me say at the outset: You can not legislate trust. You cannot legislate ethics. You cannot legislate integrity. The bureaucracy can only exhaust itself in many tangled layers of obfuscation in attempts to achieve these goals. It is quite striking that in our culture doctors must constantly attest to their trustworthiness. There are innumerable documents that require signatures to affirm compliance with bureaucratic expectations. There is the inference that the societal contract in the encounter has to be documented to assure professional behavior.

It all starts with the premise that physicians cannot be trusted. Therefore, we will have to assure our patients/clients that we are who we say we are; we have done what we say we have done and we will do what we say we will do. It's almost reminiscent of the pupil being punished and having to write on the blackboard a hundred times, "I am trustworthy."

Thus, a systemic paranoia evolves. The assumption is that somewhere, sometime the outside world is going to find out and therefore one needs to protect oneself. Documentation is a method of protection.

My father maintained his patient records on five-by-eight index cards. A visit to his office would take perhaps three to five lines of description, including the patient's vital signs and an indication of what action he prescribed. There would not be much more than a few words on the card to describe what could have taken as much as fifteen minutes in the office. The office visit could have involved a thorough discussion of the patient's illness, health history, including allergies, family and social history. The fact that it wasn't written down, does not mean that these discussions did not occur.

In 1950 there was no question of the integrity of the doctor-patient relationship. However, in 2005, if it isn't written down, it didn't happen. As a consequence our charts are now eight-by-eleven sheets of paper with myriad entry requirements to indicate what exactly occurred during the visit. These exam sheets are constantly being updated to assure that every possible parameter is annotated.

Given all this, there is still a majority of the exam that is not documented. What may not be written down are elements of the patient's history that are trying to find out about the condition of the patient in a more holistic sense. For example: Where did they go on their vacation? Did their child get into college? How do they feel about their new job?

Not documented might be observations that are sometimes subtle and lend to intuitive deductions. For example one takes notice of the patient's posture, the tone of voice, a coffee stain on a blouse, innumerable indications of the patient's general status. There is no perfect chart and there never will be. All that transpires within the appointment cannot be documented. A necessary irony, but a requirement of the healthcare industry is to attest to a variety of parameters that are an expectation of a specific service code. This code indicates an appropriate payment for that level of service. The quality of the service is assumed.

Trustworthy

Today most patients' medical charts consist of multiple entries required for different levels of exams. One of the reasons we are deluged in all of this is that third-party payers require detailed documentation of every exam to assure that the payments made to the provider were appropriate for the specific services rendered. Medical records are always subject to audit to assure compliance of services delivered as they relate to specific diagnostic codes. The more complicated the exam, the greater the charges and revenues. Sufficient data has been accumulated to render a profile of appropriateness. Time or frequency is also a feature in that repeated exams may be viewed as an aberration. Hence the evolution of "red flags" that are easily determined by statistical analysis and that require explanation. For more costly services, including surgery, pre-certification by the insurers may be required. Second opinions were, at one point, a necessary evaluation prior to approval of surgery.

All this came to fruition from an attempt at cost control on the part of the insurer. It led to an erosion of trust in the integrity of the relationship between the doctor and the patient.

In one specific case, I recommended to one of my patients that she needed cataract surgery. Her insurer required a second opinion for payment. The charge for her basic eye exam in my office was $60.00. Her second opinion exam cost much more, in the hundreds of dollars. Also included in the second opinion were procedures that were not only unnecessary, but unethical. In an attempt to validate the status of my exam, the second opinion had taken my patient down an unnecessary, wasteful and expensive road.

Veracity cannot be guaranteed. Perhaps the best test here would be the patient's own ability to assess the situation. The assumptions would be that the patient was a long-time member of the practice, that the doctor had an excellent reputation and that there was an appropriate level of trust. Bureaucracies cannot generate trust.

Most physicians belong to a medical staff of a hospital. In this relationship the hospital must be assured that the physician is appropriately trained, is licensed and is also covered by malpractice insurance. On a biannual basis, these requirements are reviewed and mandated to be current. With each passing year, this effort becomes more complicated.

This is a necessary requirement for a hospital to pass the review by the Joint Commission of Accreditation of Hospital Organizations. In and of itself that appears to be a rational way of monitoring institutions. However, over the years the increased amount of documentation to achieve this "passing grade" has become staggering. It is another symptom of the level of frailty of relationships in medicine.

The integrity and trust for a physician in the life of a hospital is a critical feature. There are first doctor-related issues that require peer review. There is a need to assess quality and to assure that the highest level of performance is maintained. Physicians need to be checked as to the quality of maintenance of their charts. There is a need to assure that all appropriate information and attestation are in place. Attestation implies that the physician assumes the responsibility of the accurateness of the record. In some cases, administrative assistants will recommend to the doctors certain changes that would improve the completeness of the record.

"Code creep" is an interesting phenomenon that occurs. Reimbursement is determined by a level of service indicated by a code. Famous for the change in Medicare function was the initiation of DRGs (Diagnostic Related Groups). This was an attempt by Medicare to reduce costs by forcing institutions to charge specific fees related to a diagnosis. This policy had a tremendous effect on hospital revenues. Over time, hospital administrators became aware that revenue enhancement could be achieved by careful study of DRGs. As an example, greater financial rewards could be gained by simply changing a code to a higher level of service, hence the term "code creep." The more complicated the bureaucracy, the more difficult it became to assure the veracity of the process. Insurers would deny payment for services and hospitals would then have to appeal their decisions. Often doctors were called in to defend, in formal testimony, the veracity of their charts. Today denials are a major element in the rationalizing of the budgetary process of hospitals and healthcare organizations.

On another level of trust, doctors involved with hospital workings were partners in the strategic planning of their institutions. Either as members of hospital boards, administrations or medical staffs, doctors were part of the team in managing long-term strategies. During the nineties, enormous pressures were developing in institution survival with healthcare organizations becoming more and more competitive.

In Philadelphia, for example, there were more hospital beds than were necessary. Some hospitals were closing, while other hospitals were merging in an attempt to survive (horizontal integration). Still others created various forms of affiliations with tertiary centers (vertical integration). In some instances, physicians gave up their autonomy to become either partners in these new arrangements or fully-employed by them. Here the relationships were transformed from a professional venue to a business connection.

In most of these cases, the relationship between the physician and the institution did not flourish and over time many actually failed. Doctors, in general, do not operate well in a business environment. Their very nature implies altruism, which is not a priority in business.

The issue of malpractice has had an extraordinary effect on the levels of trust in our healthcare delivery. Aside from the fact that there are those who have legitimate claims, the point of view of the doctor takes on a severe change. An emergency room physician told me recently that statistically he has a chance of being sued once every two years. (This is a national experience statistic for emergency room physicians.) He now approaches every patient as a potential litigant. What does this do for the trusting relationship? In my own experience, it has been the farthest thing from my mind. Perhaps it is because I enjoyed the "golden age" of medicine and this level of angst did not exist throughout my thirty years of practice. I am also fortunate that my specialty is not as high risk as some others. Specifically for an emergency room physician there is no history of doctor-patient relationship, there is no continuity. Trust is at risk when there is no continuity.

While still considering trust, let's look at a different issue. There is the public perception that patients have lost their rights in the area of healthcare. There is a belief that patients have lost their ability to determine their healthcare choices. What is interesting is that our Constitution endows us with certain inalienable rights. In other words, at one time we had rights which we now apparently are being denied and therefore we need legislation to assure that our healthcare rights are extant and not vulnerable. My question would be, what happened to those rights? Who took them away? My theory on this is related to the high level of obscuration of the interface between patient and provider. There is no longer a clear feedback system between the patients' needs and the ability of the healthcare community to respond. The more layers of bureaucracy between these elements, the more impossible the situation.

> *"The monumental transformations occurring in healthcare have been accompanied by a cacophony of discourse purporting respect for patient autonomy and commitment to patient empowerment. Frequently these are spelled out in patient's bill of rights documents. The high-sounding rhetoric goes hand in hand with the actual attenuation of these hallowed rights. Hospital ombudsmen and medical ethicists are recruited to buff the jagged edges of an impersonal system."* Bernard Lown, *The Lost Art of Healing*, 321.

Regulating Trust

Trust, in most practices, is understood and is inherently essential in the "contract" between the doctor and the patient. While outside regulations put pressure on the office environment, trust must survive. Courtesy and consideration for the values and expectations of physician and patient are a vital component of this relationship. There may be cultural differences that can be confusing. Sensitivity to the needs and expectations of others becomes more problematic in the intricacies of our healthcare culture.

Physicians, as well as their staffs, are often overwhelmed with attention to rules and regulations so that it becomes difficult to react as a human in these sensitive relationships. The new laws with regard to patient privacy, Health Insurance Portability Accountability Act (HIPAA), have put restrictions on our ability to openly communicate with our patients. Respect, courtesy, and civility are being regulated in terms of patients' rights to privacy. What would have been automatic behavior from the heart, now has to be dictated by rules and regulations

Regulations require physicians to be informed that a patient's medical information is a private issue and should be handled confidentially. Today with "privacy" being legislated, even the most compassionate behavior is restricted. These regulations place unnecessary and artificial controls on relationships.

Recently, I received a phone call from the son of an elderly patient indicating that she was going to have a problem getting to the office for an early morning appointment. The patient had just suffered a stroke and her concerned son was simply trying to make it easier for her to keep her appointment. According to the new privacy regulations, my staff cannot make any special arrangements with the son over the phone without his mother's permission. It was my job to do what had to be done to make it easier for my patient, i.e., change the appointment time.

Patients waiting in the office are theoretically not to be announced by their names when called to the exam room. The principal reason is the patient's privacy must constantly be guarded and therefore their names should not be spoken in an open waiting room. Also, computer screens are to be directed in such a way that only the receptionist can view the information. Conversation in exposed areas should be kept to a minimum with all medical information kept confidential and appropriately guarded. What used to be common sense behavior is now dictated in a series of Federal guidelines and regulations.

These continuous restrictions slowly cause a cultural change that eventually leads to a loss of directness in relationships and an increased difficulty for us to behave as the human beings that we are. It forces, to some extent, a self-conscious awareness of what the bureaucrats would determine to be inappropriate. It imposes a stilted environment in which the physician is even further challenged to try to establish or maintain the rapport that is necessary. The government cannot legislate ethics, integrity, and courtesy. By attempting to do so, obstacles are built which prevent physicians from practicing medicine as they were trained to do. Obviously, physicians and their staffs continue to operate within these laws; however, efficacy severely suffers. To successfully comply with these rules and regulations, added staff is needed, paperwork is increased, and physician-patient communication becomes a sensitive issue.

One of the most significant new additions to our office is the paper shredder. At first it was a small item, pushed in the corner. On occasion, it could be heard as it went into use. Within a few short months it was replaced with a new and larger model. Today the shredder is in operation throughout the day. We have huge collection bins which are removed by a contracted agency. Shredding has a life of its own. There is even software to take shredded material and put it back together again.

What does this say about today's society? I suppose it does have value, but there is a larger issue as to the level of paranoia that has developed.

As I treat one patient after another, I must point out the overkill in the new restrictions of the Health Insurance Portability Accountability Act (HIPAA) and other similar forms of legislation. Individually, most patients seem to see issues in the office in a forth right manner. It is the healthcare culture that seems to be moving in an overly restrictive direction.

An interesting statement by David Lilienthal suggests a concern when *"Any form of government, therefore, and any other institutions which make men means rather than ends in themselves, which exalt that state or any other institutions above the importance of men, which place arbitrary power over men as a fundamental tenet of government, are contrary to this conception; and therefore I am deeply opposed to them."*

Regulatory agencies have placed great pressure on our society. With the obvious intended benefits, there are also unintended consequences which are in some cases egregious. Each one of us is familiar with the Internal Revenue Service (IRS) and its mode of operations. In the practice of medicine we are now under the control of Medicare, Equal Employment Opportunity Commission (EEOC), Occupational Safety and Health Administration (OSHA), Environmental Protection Agency (EPA), HIPAA and others. All have the ability to scrutinize our practice, audit us, place sanctions and can do so unannounced and without warrant.

". . . irrational regulation, with its blind indifference to the relationship of costs and benefits, punishes everyone.

It is obvious that no such viciously arbitrary assault on the American productive system could occur were it not backed up by the police powers of the state. And in form, as well as in substance, the regulatory bureaucracy is dictatorial. . . The rulings of American regulatory agencies are largely unintelligible, and accordingly the American businessman is cowed into submission and a state of permanent fear. He has no way today of knowing what the law is or whether he is in compliance with it. Not only are many of these regulations self-contradictory and mutually contradictory, but they are also written by government lawyers in a

horrendous bureaucratic jargon which increases their impenetrability.
The agencies themselves cannot understand many of their own rulings."
William E. Simon, *A Time for Truth* (New York: McGraw Hill Co.,
1978), 188–189.

Concurrent with these regulatory activities is the perception that we
are guilty until proven innocent, therefore, we can be sanctioned and
then have to prove our innocence. This is similar to the IRS where you
may be audited without evidence of wrongdoing, but in direct contrast
to our jurisprudence system where you are innocent until proven otherwise.

So it is with the agencies with which we now must deal, as an audit
is required to prove that we are doing things correctly. In some cases
we are encouraged to do an internal audit, to show "good faith." If the
internal audit shows lack of compliance, then evidence of remedy must
be supplied. In one specific instance in Medicare, if an internal audit
uncovers a problem and remedies are applied with compliance not being achieved, financial compensation to Medicare may be mandated.

The rule books for Medicare, as well for OSHA, EPA and HIPAA
are massive. It is impossible for any individual or group to be in total
compliance. In our practice we have hired consultants and spent thou-
sands of dollars to not only be compliant, but more importantly, to
show good faith. Phillip Howard in his book "The Death of Common
Sense" has stated that "we are in a state of involuntary noncompli-
ance." Given the hierarchy of the regulatory agencies I can say that this
condition is permanent.

There is further purposeful obfuscation to the rhetoric of the documents that we are asked to review. This even passes down to the patients who are required to know the rules and regulations as they apply
to them. When recently introducing HIPAA to our patient groups, I was
met with glazed stares. When my staff asked patients about their "privacy rights," their response was humorous. Holding the paper their re-
ply was usually the same, "This is just another one that I have received
this week; everyone is handing them out, I don't need another one."
We then had to ask the patient to sign a document affirming that they
had been given our statement of privacy for healthcare information. In
one instance, a colleague cited that patients have now been provided a
new road map to encourage litigation.

Where does all this lead? At times I feel fortunate to be in my later years as a physician, but then I also recognize that I am about to enter those years when I am likely to be a patient. As a society, we need to be aware of the choices we make. We do have that opportunity. In government, ideas and choices can become politicized thus in time, even lose their effectiveness. As individuals we do have the privilege of relating to one another and to enjoy the God-given abilities that we own. We must, on the other hand, recognize the "loss of rights" and the "loss of freedoms" that are inherent in the layers of regulations that, while well intentioned, have in many instances lost their way in application.

". . . I ultimately realized the profundity of the difference between the businessman and the government bureaucrat. The businessman's standard of efficacy is a solution to the problem, and the more responsive he is to external reality, the better. The bureaucrat's standard of efficacy is obedience to the rules and respect for the vested interests of the hierarchy, however unyielding of a solution; response to external reality is often irrelevant." Simon, *A Time for Truth,* 55.

Intuition

"All physicians have had the experience of 'just knowing' what a diag-nosis is, with little or no information to go on. We attribute this to expe-rience, but really it's more. It's intuition." Larry Dossey, M.D., *Rein-venting Medicine (San Francisco:* Harper Collins, 1999), 25.

A good attribute for any physician is having intuition or as Webster de-fines it, "ability to know without the conscious use of reasoning." This skill, like trust, is innate. Intuition is generally not trainable, and it is cer-tainly not a course in the medical school curriculum. While intuition is not part of a didactic assessment of pre-med students in applying to med-ical school, it is a characteristic that is deemed worthy. Intuition is one of the subtle qualities that can set one physician apart from others. It can be cultivated and nurtured. Knowledge base can certainly enhance the level of intuitive behavior. I would suspect that age, to some level, increases the likelihood that intuitive judgment will be of value. Intuition, as it is in-herent, may be filtered by bias and be subjective. Intuitive thinking would then need to be assessed as to the quality of outcomes. Intuitive responses may not always be correct. The greater the history of successful intuitive responses, the more likely would be the value

Intuitive thinking uses both objective and subjective reasoning. *Beauty is in the eye of the beholder*, to cite a subjective observation. Taste is a cultural filter that affects judgment. Experience sets up a se-ries of internal flags that give direction. These and other factors will impact on intuitive responses.

Intuition is priceless. To make a medical decision, the physician must combine numerous observations and come to one solid conclusion.

Remember Mrs. Lafferty; today she is a content, functioning eighty-three year old woman with early signs of macular degeneration, a potentially blinding condition. How should she be handled?

Intuitively, one would know that she will probably live out her life with normal vision. Using my intuition, I, as her physician, should know that Mrs. Lafferty's outcome would be far more harmful, in the long-run, if I simply labeled her condition as macular degeneration and walked out of the room.

Again using my intuition, my discussions with Mrs. Lafferty should be comforting and set up a sensible strategy to monitor her disease and confirm stability; to make her feel cared for and secure.

> *"Whatever the explanation, there is absolutely no justification for assaulting patients with language that cows and disempowers. A patient must never be compelled by fear into difficult choices."* Bernard Lown, *Lost Art of Healing* (New York: Zachary, Shuster, Harmsworth Agency, 1999), 77.

Keeping in mind Dr. Lown's quotation "words can be maiming," Mrs. Lafferty's case is an ideal example of how to manage a patient using intuitive direction.

There are similar cases to which I have been exposed. During the years I have been in practice, I have acknowledged aging as a necessary consequence of staying alive. However, some of us do it better than others. It's okay to grow up; you don't have to grow old. Part of my dealing with the elderly is to acknowledge that fact of maturation in light of the privilege that long life can bring us. One of the joys of getting older is that passion for life that seems to accelerate with each year. While positive energy leads to better health, attitude leads to better outcomes.

The old adage that if you view the glass as half-full rather than half-empty you will be a happier and healthier person is certainly true. It has been my responsibility as a physician to couch opinions in such a way that a patient can find some control in the situation and see his or her personal glass as half-full. This forms to some extent my internal bias as a part of the intuitive process.

"Optimism is a Kantian moral imperative and, for the physician whose role is to affirm life, a medical imperative." Lown, *The Lost Art of Healing,* p 89.

I recently lost a patient who was in her late nineties. I had followed Mildred Simons for some thirty years and throughout this time she continued to show a progressive frailty in her eye exams. Though she barely weighed a hundred pounds, this tiny wisp of a woman was energetic and engaged in enjoying her life. And what I found amazing was that she had a memory that was more acute than many of my patients who were much younger.

Her optic nerves were paler than normal; the bulk of nerve tissue was somewhat less than I would have liked. She had had cataract surgery and had done quite well. She maintained normal visual acuity and her visual fields were normal. Once again, it was my intuitive sense that I did not have to burden her with my concerns in regard to her frailty. I chose to follow her carefully and monitor the situation.

If she had lived to 110 years, she might well have developed a problem with her eyesight. Happily, as it turned out she had normal vision to the end of her days and wasn't shadowed by the fear that she might eventually have a problem with her sight.

Perhaps we should all ask ourselves the question, "How much do any of us want to know about our physiologic future?" Technology will be offering us greater and greater ability to have this question answered. To the extent that it will improve our health there are real positive answers. With this progress will also come new questions as to our sense of well being.

We live in a culture that, while it respects the intuitive process, shows progressive desire to achieve more objectivity in decision making. I recently had an annual physical exam including a cholesterol evaluation. After the exam, I was told that taking into account my age, weight, and family history, I had a fourteen percent chance of dying within the next ten years. If I were to lower my total cholesterol below a certain level, the risk of my dying in those ten years would drop to seven percent. This statistic was determined with the use of an algorithm. Our risks in certain disease states can be ascertained to a high degree with the data that is now available.

In ophthalmology, our instruments have become so refined that we can have much better judgment on the process of change. Change is inevitable; it is the pace of change that gets our attention. When change occurs at a pace that is statistically beyond the norm, we need to have a response. Out of context, the decision might be very simple and straight forward; but put in context, it can be more complicated. Here intuitive judgment will have its value. Intuition will always have its place in medicine. Decision-making is an extraordinary process. At one end of the spectrum, a decision must be made quickly. There is no time for deliberation and consensus building. The emergency room physician seeing a patient in severe congestive failure is going to make rapid judgments and often cannot wait for laboratory studies. His actions need to be prompt, if he is to save a life.

Many medical interventions can be approached with timely deliberation. Second opinions, consultations, repeat studies can help to define the proper course of management. Here, consensus reasoning, issues of context and multiple other considerations are brought to bear. A proper direction may be reflected by a sense of comfort, or a sense of resonance. Intuition can have a place in this process. Wisdom accumulates with historical perspective and the best direction determined.

Today medicine is being shaped to favor objectivity. Practice patterns have been studied. Clinical outcomes have been assessed. Efficient, effective behavior patterns have been determined. Doctors with good clinical outcomes have been identified and their clinical pathways documented. These pathways have been presented to the physician community as preferred. The goal is to bring all doctors to the same level of clinical behavior.

Evidence-based medicine is a hot topic these days as the implication would be that better outcomes should result from such a practice imperative. Evidence based medicine relies on the premise that objective criteria are the foundation for making clinical decisions. These criteria are the result of clinical research. Better patient outcomes will result if this type of medicine is practiced.

Keeping all this in mind, the physician must always consider the patient within the context of his or her life. For example, telling a patient that the chances for complications from his or her surgery are less than one percent won't alleviate any grief if this particular patient has a poor outcome and is in that dreaded "one percent." Just such a case occurred recently with one of my patients. Jeanette Hill is in her fifties and the mother of three teenage children. Her exam revealed an advanced cataract in one eye and another one developing in the other eye. She was very upset and discouraged with her condition. I urged her to have her cataract removed and reassured her, since she did not have any complicating factors, that the surgery had a 99 percent success rate. I further explained that after the surgery she could look forward to returning to her active life. Jeanette was enthusiastic and couldn't wait to have it done. The surgery went well and she was sent home to return the next day for follow-up evaluation. That night, Mrs. Hill called the office to say that she was concerned that everything seen with the operated eye was black and questioned whether she should be able to see any light. She was asked to come to the office without delay, where it was discovered that she had a retinal detachment. It was days before Christmas, and Jeanette was admitted for emergency retina-repair. After the surgery, Mrs. Hill remembered my surgical statistic and noted that she had unfortunately fallen into that "one percent" I had previously described.

Evidence-based medicine does have its value. It is, however, equally important for the physician to remember to look at the "bigger picture" and to try to understand the circumstances in which each patient lives. Doing this takes being a good listener, having some wisdom, intuition and (most importantly) years of experience.

In the case of 83-year-old Mrs. Lafferty, her chances of developing macular degeneration are ten percent. If she is told this possible outcome without any consideration for her immediate functionality, I think she will be done a disservice.

A physician with good intuition will be more successful. The less intuitive the physician, the more anxious and dysfunctional situations with patients may become. Compassion might be interpreted as this needed quality, but, I believe, that compassion is too broad. Intuition, on the other hand, implies an understanding that goes deeper than compassion. In the clinical situation, intuition leads to a knowledge that is hard to put into words.

In one case, I was evaluating Mary Smith, an attractive, fit young woman in her twenties who had come to the office complaining of headaches. Mary's mother accompanied her to the appointment in order to drive her home after Mary had the dilating eye drops. In taking the history, Mary really had no health problems. During my evaluation, I took note she mentioned that she was going through a divorce.

As the exam progressed, every question that I asked Mary was immediately answered by her mother who was sitting off to the side. To avoid her mother responding for her, I addressed Mary and looked directly at her. Even with this tact, Mary's mother would interfere and correct her daughter or make additional comments. Within a few minutes, I was also getting a headache and intuitively knew that Mary's eye exam was probably not going to show any direct correlation to her headaches. As it turned out, I was right and Mary's eye exam was totally normal.

Since I had known the family for some time, I felt comfortable making some recommendations. First, I told Mary that her exam was normal. Secondly, I told her that this diagnosis came as no surprise to me, because after the exam, I had a headache, too. I gently explained that she needed to address several of the other problems in her life. Her headache was simply an indication or clue all was not right and she needed help to answer those questions.

> "... medicalization is the response to mounting social frustrations. Dissatisfactions with one's job or marriage or children, or with one's lot in life, are not uncommonly somaticized. Most doctors do not have the time, patience, training, or incentives to become involved in these societal quagmires, and their inattention leads patients to shop around for a quick fix. Unless they encounter an empathic physician who helps assuage symptoms, focus on the potential source of the problem, and teach them how to endure life's constraints, these troubled people increasingly turn to alternative medicine, with many falling prey to charlatans."
> Lown, *The Lost Art of Healing*, 317.

I could recount many similar stories, some with graver outcomes, but Mary's story is an example of treating the whole patient while using your experience, recognizing the context, sensing the correct direction and identifying the solution.

Headaches are ubiquitous in ophthalmology and, through my years of listening to patients' symptoms, I can say with assurance that most headaches are not caused by eye problems. However, eye exams are frequently one of the first evaluations for headaches. Headaches are extraordinarily common and patients often do not seek attention for them unless they are either out of character for their day-to-day experience or are so severe that they are interfering with their lives. The solutions are most commonly not originating from eye problems. The doctor is put in a position of rendering his best judgment as to management and the next steps. This is when a physician can really be of value to weigh the symptoms with the exam in the context of the patient's daily life.

It has been estimated that as many as sixty percent of visits to doctor offices are generated by symptoms that have no organic origin. Nevertheless, these are still symptoms, and in some cases, are believed to be urgent, if not an emergency. Acute anxiety, in its own right, can be devastating. Any symptom needs to be evaluated, because the patient's perception is the reality with which a physician has to deal.

Mrs. Jones came to the office because her eyesight had severely deteriorated. Her main complaint was that she had not been able to read a book in months. As she was in her eighties I suspected glaucoma, a cataract or retinal disease. At the outset, I established that she had 20/20 vision and her eyesight was adequate for reading. I found no pathology in the eye exam. When I went back to her medical history, and, most importantly, took the time to listen to Mrs. Jones, I learned that she liked to read in the evening after dinner. However, recently she discovered that she just couldn't stay awake.

After further conversation, I found out that her daughter had a new job and as a result, Mrs. Jones was babysitting for her two small grandchildren. At the end of the exam, I smiled and said that her only worry was that she had to make a choice between baby-sitting or reading!

The real joy in being a physician is not simply making the correct diagnosis, but correlating, to the best of your ability, what you know scientifically with what you can ascertain in the holistic sense about your patient. This results in an approach that gives the patient the tools to help control their situation. They are empowered by understanding. They are not fearful of losing control of their lives. Diagnosis, absent compassion, is harmful.

Intimacy

The extent to which a doctor and patient can share information will vary for many reasons. One patient might simply require suturing of a laceration, another removal of a corneal foreign body, thus there may be no need for any extensive involvement by the physician. However, the other extreme would be a patient who may have need of a deeper bond with the physician. Individuals may be reticent to reveal their concerns, fears or anxiety, but a physician must be sensitive to the possible need for further questioning.

The intimacy between a physician and patient implies a deeper understanding and relationship that is not seen in most professional relationships. In a medical relationship however, it is not uncommon and may be very helpful in diagnosing and suggesting corrective action. The need for intimacy may not always be obvious, but when appropriate, can be very helpful

One of the issues in our current culture has to do with the simple fact that many of us find it difficult to be intimate with ourselves. "Knowledge of self" is often illusive, if not frightening. We live in a society that is full of distractions, constantly stimulated with sounds, busy agendas and multiplicities of expectations. The mere thought that any of us have an opportunity to stop and meditate, muse about events may seem even boring to some. How much silence fills our lives? Do we even have a moment of quiet to think of our own circumstances?

"The Art of Happiness" by the Dalai Lama suggests that self-awareness can be enhanced if we have an opportunity to be silent. At the break of day each of us has some kind of schedule. The constant backdrop of sound fills our elevators, cars and every supermarket. Sound accompanies us while jogging, working on the tread mill, or while on hold on the telephone. We become uncomfortable in silence. However, it is precisely in the depths of the silence where we begin to have a sense of who we are.

Intimacy begins at home and is not always a simple process of understanding. Many of us may live for years without knowing why we conduct ourselves the way we do. Most of us have precise reactions to specific stimuli. Perhaps we find that we become irrational when angered. Some may find that they are most constructive when they are exposed to competition. Understanding ourselves will lead to self-knowledge that may help to develop secondary characteristics such as confidence, shyness, or aggressiveness. What we may not appreciate is that there can be physiologic consequences to these acts of self-knowledge.

The majority of us go through life believing we are in control of our physiologic state. Young healthy individuals cognitively feel that they are masters of their fate. And, for most of them, there is probably no reason to think that isn't the case.

Unknown to most us is the reality that primal forces control our daily life. These forces have to do with the primitive drives for survival that are a part of the deeper brain functions, are learned or inherited and are associated with hunger, pain, temperature control and what are known as "flight or fight" mechanisms. We might have a sense of fore-warning, foreboding, discomfort, or restlessness. These can be the result of a lack of congruity between what we think we perceive and what our inner-self signals as a warning. The cognitive self might be cheerfully enjoying a beautiful day while the primitive self sends out signals of warning. Often we have not the slightest idea why this sense of uneasiness is upon us.

One of the most obvious results of such uneasiness is illness. As much as we think we are in control of our lives, a lack of balance between the cognitive and deeper levels of our psyche can lead to physiologic changes. The foundation of our emotional well-being is the balance of the deeper, primitive drives and our cognitive behavior.

In the office, while I am listening to a patient's history, within moments, an obvious concern often evolves. One of the most common problems that patients bring up is their dozing or falling asleep while reading. While the patient's cognitive self says or tells him, "Time to read;" his primitive brain says, "Not on your life!"

Recently, Mr. Winter, an intense patient complained of blurred vision after reading Norman Mailer for six hours. I told him that I had the remedy and it came in the form of Norman Mailer glasses. We laughed together as we shared the obvious. I would think that anyone reading Norman Mailer for six hours should have blurred vision. The cognitive self keeps trying to drive the system when fatigue finally becomes the master. Wouldn't it be wonderful if there was such a thing as glasses to amplify anything: your golf game, your SAT scores, your bank account? Blurred vision in this case is a symptom of fatigue and not a failure of the eyes. The eyes are often the first sign of impending fatigue.

As has been said, close to sixty percent of office visits are for symptoms that have no organic basis. There are no immediate physiologic findings. Patients' symptoms are real to them. Their perceptions are their reality. They need to be treated to have a sense of return to normalcy. Doctors must understand the mechanisms behind these symptoms in order to satisfactorily manage them.

At a higher level of physiologic consequence, obesity, hypertension, headache (to name a few), can be the outcome of psychological incongruity. The body is truly a remarkable barometer. It is exquisitely sensitive to changes in emotional balance. Most of us live such a complicated existence that we are not aware of the deeper emotional drives. We need to be better at tuning into ourselves. The doctor should be in a position to help in these instances.

The role of the physician is to first diagnose, then treat. In the best of all possible worlds, the physician will have the time, the listening capacity, the interest and the desire to get the job done. In medical school, we were taught that the two toughest conditions to treat were a chronic low-grade fever and anemia. I wish it were that simple in the office setting. A thorough medical history, a complete physical exam, and laboratory studies will all lead to answers. The ability to listen is an extraordinary talent and is the most important clinical tool that a physician uses. With all its importance, the art of listening is not taught in medical school.

There are different categories of listening. First, there is listening without engagement which is modeled after Dragnet's Sergeant Joe Friday's, "Just want the facts ma'am."

Then there is listening with bias filters. In this case, the listener hears what he or she wants to hear and singles out issues that either support a preconceived notion or feed into a standard format.

Finally, there is constructive listening. Now, if one is fortunate to engage with a constructive listener, the results are magical. There is a potential for sensing at both the cognitive and emotional level that a constructive dialogue leads to discoveries, direction, diagnosis and remedies. The ability to listen constructively is truly one of the great gifts in the practice of medicine. It allows the doctor-patient relationship to take on its full meaning. It is priceless given the complicated lives and situations in which we live.

Self-knowledge is a necessary tool to appreciate a sense of personal intimacy. If one cannot be intimate with oneself, being intimate with another person will become even more difficult. A physician, in approaching a clinical issue with a patient, will find the tools of intimacy invaluable. Obviously, the physician's clinical judgment is always essential. Initially a patient may have no idea where a conversation is leading until there is a particular word used by the patient or the doctor. There may be a certain phrase, slight inflection, change in gaze, or even a shift of body that to the doctor is a vital clue.

Years of experience leads to the observation that these occasions do not occur by chance. There is a deeper mechanism controlling the event. The doctor who has the opportunity and also the ability to listen is more likely to find the right direction. This takes time, privacy, trust and intuition, a remarkable environment which can lead to the possibility of not only diagnosing and treating, but healing

Getting well, in fact healing, is a truly remarkable experience for both the physician who heals and the patient who receives the therapy. For the patient, it is not simply a sense of normal temperature, lack of pain, or loss of dizziness. It is a sense to the core that he is well. It is truly a holistic experience. Issues of illness lead to depression, fear, ignorance, and loss of control over one's life. Expectations are reduced to a life that is counted in minutes, not days. There is nothing to look forward to except day-to-day survival. There is the fear that life, as the patient knows it, will forever be changed.

In Mrs. Lafferty's case, her perception could be that all people with her ailment of macular degeneration will eventually go blind. Doctors don't have enough time to explain illness and outcomes. In many instances, they give patients a pre-printed paper that in a perfunctory way explains what is wrong with them. Today, patients surf the web and research to be absolutely certain they are at risk. They may try to obtain second opinions.

Our society is packed with information, that if we are not cautious will generate an enormous amount of paranoia and illness. Patients need a compassionate, knowledgeable listener in their physician who is prepared to answer these issues. The art of healing has to do not just with the disease we are treating, but the human being with whom we are dealing.

Patients need to feel a connection with their physicians during their medical appointments. This need is sensed by both the doctor and by the patient.

If there are any uncertainties, physicians should ask the patient, "Are there any questions or issues that we haven't covered? Are you comfortable with this direction?" For a patient, or for that matter for anyone, knowing that someone is there for you in time of need is very reassuring. Often, having a supportive family member or spouse equally informed as to the state of affairs is helpful.

Intimacy is not always a part of the clinical environment. When it is evident in difficult situations, intimacy is enormously beneficial in healing in the complete sense of the word. There is no question that healthy people are healthy because they feel well. There is a positive feedback mechanism that keeps them there. There is no question that attitude is a harbinger of wellness. There is a wonderful story of a woman who decided that she had no choice about her attitude in the book, "Fish," by Stephen Lundin, PhD., Harry Paul and John Christensen. This is a story of a woman who works in a relatively toxic office environment. She is chosen to manage an office that has a reputation for being difficult. While searching for ideas she comes in contact with the famous Pike's Seafood Market in Seattle. There she finds an extraordinary attitude towards work, if not life. She learns a new approach and takes it to her work-place. Much to the delight of all, she is successful in resolving the office dilemma. It had to do with positive energy, positive attitude. She states, "Working here has literally saved my life. It may sound sappy, but I believe I have an obligation to seek out and find ways to demonstrate my gratitude for the life I enjoy." What a marvelous testimony to attitude. If we could all find our way, this alone would lead many to health and wellness.

In some cases, I have decided that there are patients who must enjoy being miserable or unhappy or down in the dumps. I have to admit that, as hard as I try, there are times I find it difficult to successfully treat this type of pessimistic patient. Sometimes, I have actually let my frustrations be known and, interestingly, my admission has "turned the lights on" or "has opened their eyes" and suddenly our dialogue has become more productive.

True medicine, the art of healing, is in a precarious position. The "Art of Medicine" has been described as being broken. Physicians have abdicated their role as that of being healers. I have discussed three of the extraordinary tools of trust, intuition and intimacy, available to doctor and patient that enable them to have the opportunity to manage the anxiety of an illness. The practice of medicine is intriguing for the scientist in every physician, but it is through the art of healing that the doctor fulfills his real potential. Our society is moving in the direction where the traditional doctor-patient relationship is an "endangered species." And yet, this relationship is so desperately needed especially in today's cacophonic life. Good health brings with it the dividends of happier families, more productive lives, less dependency on expensive resources, and, most importantly, a positive attitude to face life's challenges.

Changes are going to occur, that is certain. There is also likely to be acceleration in the rate of change. Adaptive responses will evolve and society will move on. Healthcare will undergo similar forces. While some influences on this adaptation may be beyond our control, in other areas, we will have choices. While life can be chaotic, we do have the ability to make choices.

In structuring these choices we need to establish priorities. We need to have a hierarchy of approaches. The simplest of these choices should be to allow the doctor-patient relationship to survive and be accessible. It needs to be valued at the highest level, not only in the clinical experience, but in the medical school environment, as well. The doctor-patient relationship should not only be discussed, but also practiced, in the medical school curriculum. The concerns medical students perceive as being essential or important to their professors will be reflected in their own behavior.

Clinical practices today are so time-constrained and reflective of insurance demands that adequate opportunity for the doctor-patient relationship is not afforded. Acknowledgement of this fault and remedy must be provided. There are many issues that block this solution and that is the topic of the next chapter.

"The foremost objective of the system is cost containment, and to accomplish this, hospitals create vast bureaucracies of economic managers, accountants, and lawyers, now grown more numerous than the healthcare providers. Efficiency becomes the byword dictating homogenization in dealing with any and all patient problems. Standard clinical guidelines and computer-driven algorithms define automatic courses of action for specified diagnostic categories. Such standardization, driven largely by economics, has other putative though ancillary objectives, such as improving quality of healthcare delivery, reducing costly medical errors, minimizing unnecessary procedures, and creating uniform databases for assessing and comparing clinical outcomes. Physicians who do not adhere to the guidelines are disciplined by economic disincentives and threats of job loss. In this environment, doctors increasingly become technicians leashed to assembly lines, the aim of which is to maximize throughput." Bernard Lown, *Lost Art of Healing* (New York: Zachary, Shuster, Harmsworth Agency, 1999), 321.

Economics of Health Care

The United States has the best healthcare system in the world. Even though we've all heard the terrible stories describing the purported millions of people who lack healthcare, the truth is that any individual in our country arriving at an emergency room facility with an urgent need for care will never be turned away.

Whether it is in a major hospital setting or a physician's office, I believe that a patient's needs should be the focus. The economics can be settled later. Therefore, any patient who comes to my office with critical concerns will be seen, regardless of his or her ability to pay. This has always been and will continue to be the policy of my office.

Understandably, traditional office visits require patients to show evidence of insurance coverage, co-payments and the like. In most offices, patients are called the day before their appointment to assure they have appropriate coverage for their visit.

During the years my father practiced medicine, the economics of the doctor-patient relationship were far less complicated. It was called "fee for services." My Dad was a physician in the best of terms. He also ran his practice as a successful business. His need for an income to pay his bills was balanced both by the compassion of his services and how much patients could afford for his care. Unfortunately, this type of relationship no longer exists and yet it is one of the most sensitive economic dialogues that can occur. It has been replaced by a system of bureaucratic layers that is cumbersome, expensive and fraught with errors. These intermediaries complicate, what would otherwise be, a simple economic interchange between the physician and his or her patient.

"In the medical market place, rules imposed by third-party institutions increasingly shape medical practice." John Goodman and Gerald L. Musgrave, *Patient Power* (Washington D.C.: Cato Institute, 1994), 26.

As I look back with fondness on the golden age of medicine, I recognize that there is an essential element that is critical to saving our healthcare culture. This element is self-determination.

Our society is being propelled in the direction of individuals not being involved in decision-making processes, particularly in healthcare. As one generation passes on to the next, attitudinal shifts can be recognized. Reading Tom Brokaw's book, "The Greatest Generation," you readily appreciate those who were raised during the Depression and grew up through World War II. The American work ethic was valued. Loyalty was not only an individual characteristic, but also part of institutional life. A sense of entitlement was not as evident as it is today. There was also a sense of humility and most of all deep gratitude for what this country represented.

As the economy struggled through the 1940s, employers, under pressure with wage increases, came upon the idea of substituting benefits for wages. Healthcare was one of those benefits. The advantage for the employer was that this benefit would be paid for by pre-tax dollars and therefore would be far less expensive than if the employee had purchased the same level of benefit. Thus the concept of third-party-pay was born.

From that moment on, the healthcare system of this country began a three-way conversation (patient/provider/insurer). Reminiscent of those first gray clouds on a sunny morning, there were rumblings of things to come. Initially, the plan was a good idea. The country was recovering from a war, the economy was just getting under way and what a ground-breaking notion it was to offer workers support for their healthcare through a company-supported program. While this concept was innovative, it also led in the direct loss of self-determination. From this moment on, there would be less involvement of the individual in the decision-making process for his or her health future.

"Healthcare costs cannot be controlled unless we empower individuals and make it in their self interest to become prudent buyers of healthcare." Goodman and Musgrave, *Patient Power*, 49.

Third-party-pay shifted the exchange of ideas from the once private relationship between the doctor and patient and introduced dialogues between doctor/insurance, insurance/employer, employer/employee, employee/insurance and employee/doctor. In any one-on-one relationship there is a much greater chance for success than in multiple layers of bureaucrats. There is an exponential increase in the chance of error. The consequence of error is tragic.

Perhaps you are familiar with the fact that if you are without medical insurance and have to be admitted to a hospital you will be responsible for the "whole" bill. An insured patient will be covered at a discounted rate by his insurance company. The actual dollar amount is far less than the billed amount. The uninsured will be responsible for the full amount of the bill which can be enormous. This seems a perverse situation.

Similarly, patients who are eligible for Medicaid often do not enroll. When they enter the hospital it is likely that their bills will not be paid and the institution will absorb the loss. The only interest in paying the bill comes from hospital administrators who know the likely outcome. Patients often seem not concerned. As a result the hospital staff will make it a point to try to enroll the patient in Medicaid. This would seem a peculiar function for hospital employees.

When Medicare joined the healthcare insurance system it was a great service to our senior population. It did, however, also add to further separation of the patient from the doctor through the economics of third-party-pay. Physician's fees were no longer set to the patient's ability to pay, as they were during my Dad's day, but to the amount the insurer could compensate. Patient pressure on doctors' fees was not evident and the only demand that was felt was from the sometimes negative reaction from the insurers. These were actually good times for doctors and hospitals who were both being paid for services, in many cases, for the first time.

In my own experience, in the late 1960s cataract surgery cost $400 for the surgeon's fees. In the late 1970's and the early 1980's cataract surgery fees reached as high as $4000. The only economic demand on fees was what the insurer was willing to pay. This influenced hospital fees, as well. There was also an increase in administration as more paper work was involved. Whole new process flows were a concomitant of Medicare. The architecture of our hospitals changed to afford the requirement for larger office-space. In many hospitals patient beds were replaced with business space. Upper management boomed. Vice Presidents were ubiquitous.

These new economics of healthcare brought about change in patient attitudes. At first it may have seemed all this was a wonderful new direction, almost a gift. There was a sense of relief which was followed with a sense of expectation that now has progressed to a sense of entitlement. Today we have no economic dialogue between the doctor (now considered the provider) and the patient (now considered the client). The actual visit to the doctor's office is labeled an encounter.

In Barbara Tuchman's book entitled "The March of Folly," she describes folly as a course of action people take knowing full well that what they are doing is wrong. It is the decision of a group of people to pursue a policy that is contrary to self-interest. The book describes several historical events in the light of this theory. Governmental decisions are prone to miscalculation. History is full of such events. In the healthcare system we are following, we seem to passively accept third-party intervention as the only solution to our dilemma.

It is remarkable that as a society, we continue to proceed with our healthcare system regardless of all the evidence that's stacked against it. The only answers that we find are increased bureaucracy. The layers of regulations are becoming suffocating, not only for the physicians, but for the patients, too. The product of the industry is the ability of the doctor to deliver services to the patient. If you hypothetically remove the doctor and patient out of the equation what remains? You are left with an enormous, expensive bureaucracy.

Interestingly there are doctors and patients doing just that. They are exiting the system. Many areas of our country now have physicians practicing proprietary medicine in which the doctor and patient determine the value of services. The physician offers a contract to care for a patient for a specific period of time. The physician guarantees access, but requires payment up front for that period of service. The relationship between physician and patient is much more direct and there is no intermediary. Fees are determined by the ability to establish enough business to meet the doctor's expectations. This solution guarantees that the patient will not only have access to a physician with whom he or she is comfortable, but it will also nurture any dialogue between the two the parties which is critical. What seems to be inherent in this system is responsible decision making by the individuals who are accountable for the choices they make. This is a central principle for the development of a rational healthcare system.

There is no nation that can afford the healthcare that is potentially available for its citizens. It's a simple fact that this country does not have the resources to pay for all the myriad health services that a population might require. Nor can any other nation do so. The obvious result is that every healthcare need cannot be met.

Healthcare costs now are exceeding fifteen percent of the gross national product. It is expected that it will increase and eventually be greater than twenty percent. Driving this progression are forces of demographics and technology. The fastest growing element of our population is our senior citizens. They are also the neediest. This will have an enormous effect with the coming of age of the baby boomers. Technologic and pharmaceutical advances, while greatly appreciated, will compound the costs. These forces need to be reconciled.

Managed-care has been one of the recent tools to control the use of resources while still operating within free market principles. Employers purchase programs for their employees who enroll in Health Maintenance Organizations (HMO). There are a variety of choices; one of the more popular at this time is the Preferred Provider Organization (PPO). Managed-care organizations operate with internal methods to control access as well as costs. This approach has been successful in controlling costs in the recent past. At this time, however, it is no longer able to maintain the explosion of healthcare costs.

Physicians are encouraged to comply with the objectives of managed-care organizations. Peer review attempts to set standards of utilization. Physicians are financially credentialed. For example, a physician whose practice is focused on senior care is more likely to have higher costs of operation. This is a less attractive practice for a managed-care group. Greater margins are achieved with practice groups involving younger patients. Any practice, even pediatrics, that focuses on high-risk cases is difficult to include in a managed-care organization.

Physicians have different styles in their approach to practicing medicine. In some cases their methods are much too expensive to support the system. Physician behavior is advised by their colleagues. Preferred practice patterns are suggested and, if acknowledged, an attempt is made by the physician to change the style of the practice. These suggested changes can alter studies ordered, therapeutic strategies considered, medications prescribed (such as generics), and even the amount of time spent with each patient. In employment models, physicians were clearly seen to be less productive. Goals had to be set. Many physicians became disillusioned by these methods.

While for a decade the acceleration of healthcare costs was controlled by the introduction of managed-care, the honeymoon for our society is over. Healthcare costs will now go through acceleration. Providers have been pushed to the point of going out of business. There is little margin for hospitals to have access to capital. Infrastructure cannot be maintained. Institutions cannot provide cutting-edge technology if they have no capital. Physicians' offices have also been pushed to the limit. Particularly in the higher risk specialties of obstetrics, orthopedics and neurosurgery growth has been stilted by the high costs of malpractice. Younger doctors are prone to choose less risky specialties. Senior physicians are finding it difficult to stay in practice when it is so expensive to maintain such insurance. The very litigious nature of our culture forces older doctors to wonder why they should work in such a high risk environment.

There is also the issue of the repayment of medical school loans. Many young physicians are in debt in excess of $100,000. This is an enormous burden in terms of their economic freedom and also what choices they can make. They are forced to enter group practices or partnerships where they have a guaranteed salary. Gone are the days of the "neighborhood doc" hanging up his shingle. The experience of both debt and malpractice have a tremendous effect on the attitude and ultimate behavior of new physicians. The altruism of the medical school environment can be quickly changed to cynicism if not thoughtful. There is a sense of loss of control of one's professional life.

Hospital and physician practices have attempted to affect revenue flow to their offices by having in-house managers review diagnostic and billing codes. There is an attempt to assure payment by keeping accurate records. Denial of payments has been an ongoing problem, particularly for hospitals. Appeals are frequent. This is all time consuming and expensive.

Federal and state laws can change relatively abruptly and seriously affect the way healthcare facilities strategize. A five-year plan would seem impossible in this environment. Building codes can be changed having a tremendous effect on the plans of old and new construction. The straight forward improvement of technology is not as serpentine as bureaucratic proliferation. Doctors and hospitals have a compelling need to move in the direction of improved services for their patients. This becomes exquisitely difficult in this environment.

The pharmaceutical world is increasingly becoming ensnarled in the world of bureaucracy. The patient is no longer the buyer of pharmaceutical products; the buyers of drugs today are becoming larger groups. The ones making the economic choices today are managed care entities and Pharmacy Benefit Managers (PBM). The purchase of pharmaceutical products is now through an intermediary who makes decisions as to cost and quality. The patient eventually gets the product but only after it has been scrutinized by larger organizations and determined to be a tier one, two or three product as provided in an insurance program.

Of great interest is the fact that the Federal government will become perhaps the biggest customer. If one looks at the debate in Congress as to the Medicare Pharmaceutical Benefit program, one has an insight into the dialogue that evolves about our healthcare delivery. On the liberal side is the concern for more governmental support of drug expenses for our elderly population. The more conservative side argues for the use of the open market-place to keep costs in balance. Politics and perception cast their spell as either side argues both out of conviction and a concern for their constituencies. The drama of democracy leads to a vote and decision. The outcome seems anything but simple. For example, in the proposed government program a patient pays a premium ($35/mo), has a deductible ($275), has 75% coverage up to a specific amount (here $2250), pays full price up to a second point (here

$3600) then pays only 5% beyond for as much as is required. This is your government working for you.

The patient and his/her need for pharmaceutical products are being separated by a complicated layer of politics and bureaucracy. There is no question of the need for patients to have the products that are necessary. The consequences of these complicated policy decisions only make the economics harder to resolve. Further, while the framework of the new Medicare law is that of a benefit to our elder citizens, the eventual perception is that this will be viewed as an entitlement. Consequently this pattern lends to the increasing costs of healthcare.

No one denies that senior citizens have the need for pharmaceuticals. It should be questioned whether it is the obligation of our society to foot the bill. Current Medicare law is an attempt to provide the support while still requiring some accountability on the part of the patient. Unfortunately the new Medicare pharmacy bill is enormously complicated.

Our society is losing its ability to value service. I think we all recognize service and crave it. We don't have the personal leverage to eek it out of the organizations that provide us our healthcare. The layers of management, and the endless rules make it difficult to know how to effect change. Individuals can show preference through their votes, their use of their monies or they can walk. The larger the organizations we deal with, the less likely the individual is to be successful. Bureaucracies are not in the business of service. Their goals are compliance with regulation. They have a life unto themselves. Their raison d'etre is to increase the perceived need for the society they serve. The regulations change annually. Constant vigilance is necessary to be compliant. Individuals are overwhelmed. We need to address this problem by allowing the individual's needs to be addressed. This can only occur in a more responsive setting. If the relationship between the provider and the client is direct there is a chance that service issues can be resolved. Without the clarity of the relationship, we are lost in an obscuration of details.

There are other signs of our health system struggling. Our elder citizens are going to Canada to save money by purchasing their prescriptions there. The controls on generics and pharmaceutical plans still do not offer the economic levels that they need. This picture will probably not see immediate improvement.

An attempt by Hillary Clinton to design healthcare reform was so complex that it fell of its own weight. There did not seem to be full partnership with those that were selected to do the work and those that were involved in day-to-day healthcare services. The eventual design was so complex it did not seem feasible.

Government seems more likely to impede rather than to facilitate the delivery of healthcare. One flagrant example of governmental obstruction is the tax inequity to purchasing healthcare. While employers can use pre-tax dollars to purchase healthcare insurance, individual buyers cannot. If this inequality could be resolved, it would allow individuals to buy their own healthcare policies with pretax dollars. The fact that this inequity exists forces the market-place to compete with employers, and not their employees. Employees are removed from the economic exchange and therefore their choices are limited to those of their employer. If employees were enabled to exercise their choice in the healthcare system we would be in a better position. Healthcare premiums should be tax deductible. Medicare coinsurance should also be tax deductible.

The more the market place is controlled by governmental bureaucracy the more information will be controlled by these organizations. If personal choice is a greater aspect of the system, information will be more likely to be accessible by the individual. Information and choice are critical elements in the ability of the individual to engage in the healthcare system. The more obscure the data, the less likely the individual can make educated decisions. Data has been available in managed care but in some cases it is not as accessible as it needs to be. This should be a priority. The purchase of managed care programs should be dependent to a great degree on access of data. The more obscure the costs of services, the less accurate the use of resources. While this is important to the individual, it is even more important to the doctor and insurer. Even in these latter cases, data is sometimes difficult to assess.

Most medical information is also time-sensitive. Healthcare decisions and strategies need timely considerations. Within the managed care arena, reconciliation of contracts is very difficult. The efficiency of a managed care program is to a large degree dependent on the financial feasibility of the contracts with which it is involved. Simply stated, does the percentage of premium given to the healthcare system cover the costs of providing the care? This is the objective of the managed care program, i.e., to have a surplus at the end of the contract period. However, at the end of the contract year, not all expenses are in; there are still expenses that have not been reported to the healthcare system. These are called "incurred but not reported" (IBNR) expenses. Final reconciliation of the contract cannot be completed until all expenses are in. Experience has shown that this takes thirteen months after the end of the contract year. There are actuarial predictions on these numbers but the point is that, in terms of planning, it is extraordinarily difficult to get it right. If there is a deficit, it is not a happy outcome. Deficit is difficult to manage. The choices are curtailment of services. This is extremely troublesome as it can be a quality issue. Other choices could be higher premiums for patients, less income for doctors and finally less margin to run hospitals.

In *"Patient Power"* by John Goodman and Gerald Musgrave it is pointed out that the bureaucracy suppresses individual behavior. Individual behavior is precisely what keeps a market activity rational. The more obscure, the more obfuscation, the less data, the less likely that the market will be able to correct inequities. The more attenuated the relationship between the provider and the consumer the greater the loss of efficiency in decision-making.

Individuals promote common sense; bureaucracies do not. In the past physicians were accountable only to their patients; today they are not only answerable to their patients but they are also accountable, auditable and must be in compliance with the regulations of the Internal Revenue Service, Medicare, Medicaid, Environmental Protection Agency (EPA), Occupational Safety and Health Administration (OSHA), Equal Employment Opportunity Commission (EEOC) and Health Insurance Portability Accountability Act (HIPAA), to name a few.

In Phillip Howard's book, "The Death of Common Sense," he writes that we are deluged with so many laws that we can barely keep up. Considering the number of regulations, it is probable that at any one time it is impossible to be in compliance. I have to admit that puts me in a state of perpetual involuntary non-compliance. What is shocking to realize is that a regulator can come to my office and, depending on his attitude, find that I am not in compliance and put a lock on the door.

Thus has bureaucracy controlled my behavior, as well as that of my patients.

Things aren't getting any better. We do not seem to be able to get off of this governmental merry-go-round, nor have we considered the politics of these activities. Now we are dealing with issues of principle verses coercion. David Stockman, in his book "The Triumph of Politics" gives great insight into the forces within our government that take great ideas and politicize them. What comes out is something that is hardly recognizable. If one could have faith that a government could run a free market then maybe we could rest. It seems obvious that it cannot.

History has been very clear. There have been advantages to health-care delivery with social systems that have evolved since the forties. There are consequences, however, that are taking over our ability to keep a rational healthcare system functional. The breakdown is becoming more obvious every year. It is time to recognize that it is not the government that is going to correct this situation. What is needed is to allow the free market to have its influence over a majority of healthcare delivery. In the coming years there will be great pressure on moving our country to a universal healthcare system. It will be the politically correct position to espouse such a program. In a sense it seems to be for some a "no-brainer." Precisely that, it is a no-brainer. It is easy to conjure that the government can answer all these issues. Having pointed out where we have been and our current crisis in medicine, I think that the market place is where the rational solutions lie.

As our health services increase and medical technology expands, our inability to pay for healthcare will continue to escalate. In an open market, choices can be made and in the process of choosing, value is determined. It is the perception of "value for cost" that establishes the need for a service.

Using the Adam Smith analysis of economics, the market-place gives direction to dialogue between supply and demand. It is a balanced method of rationing. If we recognize the initial premise that we can't afford the available medical services, then we must accept that there needs to be a constraint mechanism.

Some examples of resource control are portraits of bureaucratic complexity. One is to define payment for physician services in units of work. In 1992, Medicare significantly changed the means by which physicians are reimbursed for services. In place of basing physicians' payments on fee for services, Medicare instituted a standardized payment program established on resource-based relative value scale (RBRVS). The attempt was to define a unit of work and the resources required to produce that unit. All other services were then compared to this "bench mark" and paid on a relative value scale. The costs of that unit of work were related to physician effort, practice expense and professional liability insurance. Payments are calculated by multiplying the combined costs of the service by a conversion factor determined by the Center for Medical Services (CMS). Payments are also adjusted for variation in geographic differences in costs.

In a totally different sphere of influence, here is an example of service utilization that could be called rationing, but is a serious effort to define relative utility of services in the face of finite resources. In an attempt to more effectively utilize healthcare resources, Brown, Brown, Sharma and Landy, (Healthcare Economic Analysis and Value Based Medicine), Survey of Ophthalmology, 2003, have forwarded a complex system of utility analysis. Utility analysis "is the quantitative measurement of subjects' preferences regarding the quality of life associated with a particular health state." It attempts to quantify that state of health and gives it a utility value. In a perfect state of health the utility value is 1.0. Values less than 1.0 are less preferred. Interventions can then be measured by an improved state of health and given a value on this scale. The improved state of health measured on this scale can then be further characterized by the number of years associated with this state. This is called quality adjusted life year (QALY). *"The benefit of using QALYs is easily seen. They quantify the value of healthcare interventions with measures that are broad enough not to miss major issues, and allow a comparison of interventions across disparate health conditions. When amalgamated with costs, they form the basis of value-based medicine, the measure of value of healthcare received for the resources expended."*

This is an excellent attempt to deal with current issues that are unsustainable in healthcare financing. However it is enormously complex and would be difficult to implement. Its goal is not "service rendered" to the patient, but more to facilitate the effectiveness of a bureaucracy.

As has been said before, "Statistics deal with populations, doctors treat patients." It is a different form of rationing. Uwe Reinhart, the Princeton economist, has forwarded the thought that fee for services is a form of rationing. Rationing is a pejorative. Rationing is a bureaucratic process; choice is a decision by an individual. William Simon has thoughts as to the operation of a free market where choices are shaped by value and resources.

> *"It works as follows: Day in and day out, people engage in economic activities called businesses—small individual ones and gigantic ones held together by a tissue of voluntary individual contracts. They organize and allocate resources by selling and buying in markets which respond sensitively to the wishes of individuals. Each consumer "votes," in effect, with his dollar in untold thousands of market "elections," and his vote is automatically translated into shifts of resources into the desired products and services. The products for which people are willing to pay an adequate price are produced; things for which people are not willing to pay an adequate price are not produced."* Simon, *Time for Truth*, 23.

In an Adam Smith, laissez-faire open market, individuals, rather than the bureaucracy, make choices. These choices are the most clear and simple way to approach the problem, because only individuals can satisfactorily judge their own resources and opportunities.

> *"The message coming to our shores from virtually every corner of the globe is free markets work and socialism, collectivism, and bureaucracies do not. For the most part, Americans welcome that message. But in the area of healthcare, the message is falling on deaf ears. In a market system, the pursuit of self-interest is usually consistent with social goals. When an individual pursues his own interest, his actions usually benefit others as well. Precisely the reverse is true in bureaucratic, nonmarket systems. The hallmark of bureaucratic thinking is the belief that the individuals don't matter."* John Goodman and Gerald L. Musgrave, *Patient Power* (Washington D.C.: Cato Institute, 1994), 111.

Undoubtedly we are at a time in medicine where some services are considered extraordinarily expensive. In these cases the average patient would be unable to afford such care. In situations of such enormity, insurance should be considered a necessary element in payment strategy. Actuarial experience for different income levels could determine the reasonable level of protection that an individual would need.

Also to be considered in this equation are the uninsured and the disabled who would need to have support. This should come from governmental plans with the levels of applicability to be determined.

The bulk of healthcare bills would be open to choices made in the open market. This would allow the economic dialogue between the patient and the supplier to have its greatest economic effect. This would allow self determination instead of bureaucratic dictation.

The downside to this argument would be that individuals would feel deprived if they couldn't have everything they wanted. Patients would have to prioritize their decisions based on need, resource and access. This would be a difficult change. Today's patients perceive that they are entitled to any medical service they deem to be necessary. This attitude will not change until it is superimposed on the fact that resources are finite.

In our current culture the limit of resources in healthcare is manifest to the patient in such ways as referral, co-pay, deductibles, tiered pharmacy programs, limited choice, to name a few. The patient has little ability to change the behavior of insurers and managed care programs. They can choose other programs, but then this has had little effect. In a similar fashion physicians have little ability to change the behavior of insurers. In some communities there is a virtual monopoly of insurers and therefore even less economic dialogue. This only encourages an imbalance between resources and services.

Every element of the healthcare system (patients, doctors, insurers, institutions) is frail in the means in which it operates. Patients do not have a sense of accountability. Their health insurance is used for routine healthcare, as well as for more serious conditions. In contrast, most family insurance such as automobile, home, or even travel is associated with unusual occurrences.

Physicians codify their services, thus they may be encouraged to misrepresent clinical situations to enable patients to have access when they would otherwise be denied. Codification is a talent, as there is always an interest to maximize revenue. "Code creep" is a common experience in both medical practices, as well as hospital records. Ever since Diagnosis Related Groups (DRGs) were instituted by Medicare in the seventies and eighties there have been efforts by providers to enhance their productivity by the right choice of activity level. DRGs were the attempt of Medicare to facilitate the payment for given levels of service. It was successful in curtailing "run away" expenses. In response, however, providers learned how to maximize the system. This led to denials by payers to their providers and yet more bureaucratic headaches.

Insurers try to increase their market-share position by promising services to their constituents, only to drop these services at a later date if they can't maintain satisfactory margin. For every premium dollar spent on heath care, some 20–30% is kept by the insurer. Only 70–80% goes to paying for healthcare services. Most patients do not know the rules and policies of their health plans. There is purposeful obfuscation. A major part of the problem is that insurers sell their products to employers and not to individuals. The choices are made by the employer who is dictated by his own bottom line.

Dysfunctional behavior on the part of the government is partially to blame. We are a nation that supports less government intrusion in our private affairs. Self-interest is perverted in the government to become political interest. In this scheme interests of others are supported to the detriment of others. Pure self-interest works in a totally different fashion such that each participant benefits equally. The economics of healthcare do not lend themselves to political discourse.

> *"Pursuit of self-interest, then, is much more than a natural characteristic of human behavior. In most institutional settings, it is a survival requirement. The institutional setting, however, determines whether our pursuit of self-interest is primarily beneficial or harmful to others. In regulated markets dominated by bureaucratic institutions, the interest of individuals frequently conflict. One person's gain is another's loss. In such an environment, when others pursue their interests, you and I are often made worse off.*
>
> *Quite a different result emerges in competitive markets with clearly defined private property rights and individual freedom of choice. In that environment, you and I cannot pursue our own interests (for the most part) without creating benefits for others. Conversely, others rarely can pursue their interests without creating benefits for us."* Goodman and Musgrave, *Patient Power,* 13.

The only answer to this mayhem is to put individuals into a position of power of choice and allow them to make their own decisions in the market-place.

This simple step is the solution to the increasing dissonance that we hear around us. David Reisman in his book "The Lonely Crowd" asks if our society is capable of this level of responsibility. Written in 1961, Mr. Reisman's book discusses the change of moral center in our culture. He points out that earlier generations lived on a set of principles that were dominantly internal, set by their families and their heritage. Moral direction, he observes, is moving to external sources, principles that are portrayed by peer groups. There is a moral relativism. The question is has our society moved so far in this direction that it is no longer the place of the individual to accept responsibility for the choices made?

If the healthcare system is to thrive, individual choice is the critical feature. Therefore, the responsibility for making that choice and the consequences after the choice is made must be accepted by the individual. Our only recourse is in the power of the individual.

Epilogue

Mrs. Lafferty and I have had an open doctor-patient relationship for over a decade. I am delighted to say that, as I write the last pages of this book, she is a lively 93 year-old in good health who resides on her own and continues to drive. Recently, Mrs. Lafferty was in my office for her annual appointment. I am pleased to report that her vision remains satisfactory and she has never developed macular degeneration.

Mrs. Lafferty recognizes that life offers no guarantees—especially when it comes to her health. However, I have always believed that it's her positive attitude that has helped her adjust so well to all the "ups and downs" that life presents. And most importantly to Mrs. Lafferty, she knows that she can always count on me and our office for support. It has been my hope that by not burdening her with warnings of possible blindness she would retain her up-beat manner.

I have used Mrs. Lafferty as an example in my book, because I am proud of the relationship that she and I have fostered. This is one of the main reasons I took the Hippocratic oath and became a physician. As my grandfather and father before me, I wanted to give my patients a sense that their health mattered to me.

In writing *The Laying On Of Hands*, I wanted to address three main issues. The first is my overriding concern for the loss of the art of medicine. In this high-tech world of palm pilots and picture phones, our foremost goal as physicians, which is to care about our patients, must be improved. Secondly, with specific reference to macular degeneration, I wanted to point out the complexity of decision making in a frightened population when outcomes are difficult to assess and resource consumption is enormous. Finally, how does this reflect in the medical hierarchy in which we live?

All three involve change in a vibrant time of our history. All three can be examined from an exciting, positive perspective. We are blessed with the knowledge of history to help us make choices. We must resist being overcome with the frustration of failure and see the advantages of learning. We do have the benefit of making choices. We are also blessed with the enthusiasm and intelligence of our next generation medical community that is drawn to this service by the best of motivations. We live in a time where our research has been able to push back the barriers of aging. We have developed techniques of therapeutic clinical trials which help us to make clear, rational decisions in medical and surgical management. We live in the most prosperous times that man has known. We have the ability to exchange information through instantaneous communication. Within our life time we will be able to see the improved health of third-world countries. There is a positive momentum in all these themes. What is needed is the ability to articulate the principles of this momentum and to implement action plans as the way opens. Politics may rear its ugly head but principled behavior will survive, if the leadership is strong. Resources will dictate each step of the way. This is an extraordinary time and we are fortunate to be participants.

The keystone for building the bridge to health in the broadest sense is the doctor-patient relationship. The absence of this bond can only lead to isolation and alienation for the patient, and the art of medicine would vanish. This book is a testimony to the mandate of caring. We need to go beyond disease and engage in the total human being and the quest for healing.

Notes

PRACTICAL LESSONS

1. Bill Moyers, *Healing and the Mind: Public Affairs Television*, David Grubins Productions, Inc. 1993.

MACULAR DEGENERATION

2. J. Seddon, Cote, Rosner, *Progression of Age-Related Macular Degeneration*, Archives of Ophthalmology 121: 2003, 1728.

3. McGinley, Laurie, "Blindsided: Medicare Flip-Flop On Eye Drug Roils Elderly Victims-Visudyne May Ease Vision Loss, But Miscues and Mistrust Derail Government Backing-Protest by the Gray Panthers," The Wall Street Journal, July 16, 2002.

4. Editor, "Experts and the Drug Industry," *New York Times,* March 4, 2005.

Bibliography

Brown, M.D.,M.N., M.B.A., Melissa, Gary Brown, M.D., M.B.A., Sanday Sharma, M.D., MSc, M.B.A., and Jennifer Landy, M.D. *Healthcare Economic Analyses and Value Based Medicine*. Survey of Ophthalmology: Vol. 48, Number 2, March–April 2003.

Burns, Lawton R. and Wharton School Colleagues. *The Healthcare Value Chain* San Francisco, CA.: Jossey-Bass, A Wiley Company, 2002.

Dossey, M.D., Larry. *Reinventing Medicine*. San Francisco, CA.: Harper Collins, 1999.

Goodman, John C., and Gerald L. Musgrave. *Patient Power*. Washington, D.C.:Cato Institute, 1994.

Howard, Philip K. *The Death of Common Sense*. New York: Random House, 1994.

Klein, M.D., Ronald, Barbara E. Klein, M.D., Sandra C. Tomany, M.S., Stacy M. Meuer, B.S., Guan-Hua Huang, PhD. *Ten Year Incidence and Progression of Age-Related Maculopathy: The Beaver Dam Eye Study*. Ophthalmology: Vol. 109, Number 10, October 2002.

Lama, Dalai and Howard C. Cutler, M.D. *The Art of Happiness* New York: Riverhead Books, 1998.

Lundin, PhD., Harry Paul and John Christensen. *Fish*. New York: Hyperion, 2000.

Lown, M.D., Bernard. *The Lost Art of Healing*. New York: Zachary, Shuster, Harmsworth Agency, 1999.

Magee, M.D., Mike, and Michael D'Antonio. *The Best Medicine* New York: Dystel & Gooderich Lit. Mgmt., 1999.

Moyers, Bill. *Healing and the Mind*. New York: Doubleday, 1993.

Riesman, David. *The Lonely Crowd*. New Haven: Yale University Press, 1961.

Seddon, J.M., J. Cote, B. Rosner, *Progression of Age-Related Macular Degeneration: Association with Dietary Fat, Transunsaturated Fat, Nuts and Fish Intake,* (Harvard Medical School, Boston), Archives of Ophthalmology, 121: 2003, p. 1728–1737.

Stockman, David A. *The Triumph of Politics* New York: Avon Books, 1986.

Simon, William. *A Time for Truth*. New York: McGraw-Hill Company, 1978.

Sternberg, M.D., Lewis. *Photodynamic Therapy of Age Related Macular Degeneration: A Candid Appraisal*. American Journal of Ophthalmology, Vol. 137, No. 3, March 2004.

Tuchman, Barbara. *The March of Folly*. New York: Alfred A. Knopf, Inc., 1984.